The Lazy
Person's
Guide!

P9-DGC-390

Stress

Other titles in this series:

Stress

Theresa Francis-Cheung

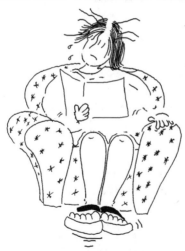

Newleaf

Newleaf

an imprint of
Gill & Macmillan Ltd
Hume Avenue
Park West
Dublin 12
with associated companies throughout the world
www.gillmacmillan.ie

© Theresa Francis-Cheung 2002
0 7171 3332 X
Design by Vermillion Design
Illustration by Emma Eustace
Print origination by Linda Kelly
Printed by ColourBooks Ltd, Dublin

This book is typeset in Rotis Semi-Sans 10pt on 13pt.

The paper used in this book comes from the wood pulp of managed forests. For every tree felled, at least one tree is planted, thereby renewing natural resources.

A CIP catalogue record for this book is available from the British Library.

5 4 3 2 1

CONTENTS

INTRODUCTION

'I'm not stressed out, I'm not, I'm not, I'm not.'

There are hundreds of books on stress and stress management, so why read this one?

1. Because it's a lazy guide. You won't have to plough through pages and pages of interesting, but often useless, information. You'll just get the information and advice you need.

2. Because the focus isn't just on major stressors, such as divorce, debt, death of a loved one, illness or a busy demanding schedule. The book also deals with life's daily frustrations, such as forgetting where you put your car keys or finding empty milk cartons in the fridge, and the important but often overlooked part they play in creating stress.

3. Because this book won't ask the impossible from you. It doesn't endorse the 'stress is bad for you and you must do everything you can to avoid it' mantra. Instead, you will learn that you can't and indeed shouldn't avoid stress; you just need to learn how to handle it.

4. Because the book assesses therapies and stress management techniques from a lay person's point of view. It answers the questions: 'Is there a point to all this?' and 'Will it work for me?'

5. Because the book encourages you to become your own stress expert. It isn't complicated or difficult to manage stress. In most instances you don't need to consult doctors, therapists, stress consultants, and self-help gurus. You don't need to

totally change your lifestyle, start meditating, take up yoga, listen to relaxation tapes or take pills and apply lotions. All you need to do is apply the simple, practical guidelines given in this book to your daily life.

At last – a realistic, accessible guide to help you live successfully with stress. I can't promise that you'll be an oasis of calm and contentment when you finish reading this book, but I can promise you that the advice here will help you keep your cool when tension mounts.

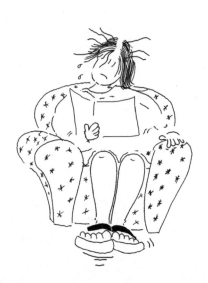

CHAPTER 1

THE MANY FACES OF STRESS

Do you worry a lot? Do you feel tired, or on edge? Are you lacking energy or suffering more aches, pains, colds and flu? Or do you feel that your life is spiralling out of control?

A yes to any of these questions could be a sign of stress.

We tend to associate stress with busy, pressured people: the overstretched parent, the high-powered executive, the student facing exams, the celebrity coping with fame and so on. But you don't need to have a busy, hectic lifestyle to feel stressed. Regardless of who you are, and what the demands on your time and energy are, everyone has to deal with stress and the effect it has on physical, mental and emotional health.

WHAT IS STRESS?

Sounds like a stupid question. It's obvious what stress is. But if you actually think about it, stress is quite hard to define. That's because stress has many faces. It means different things to different people and affects people in different ways.

It may appear that your rich, retired uncle has a stress-free life, but in fact he may be stressed by anxieties about his health, safety and a million other – as it seems to you – trivial concerns. On the other hand, the busy working mum with five children and two ex-husbands may take everything in her stride.

Pressure, tension, anxiety, doing too much, feeling out of

control, over-committing yourself, feeling threatened, living on the edge and not being able to cope all spring to mind when we try to define stress. Yet they don't take into account the fact that stress can be a good thing as well as a bad thing. Weddings, holidays, Christmas and even winning the lottery can be stressful, but in a pleasant, invigorating way.

You may wonder how positive change, such as getting married or suddenly getting rich, can be stressful. These things can be stressful because they involve change. Routines built up for years have to be replaced with new rituals, and it can be difficult to adjust to new circumstances, however pleasant they may appear to be.

So here is a definition of stress that covers both its positive and negative aspects: stress is how your body and mind react to change.

The key issue here is how you adapt to that change or how you perceive an event. If you can adjust well to the circumstances in your life, stress isn't a problem. It is when you can't adjust, or don't want to adjust, that stress causes problems. In short, it's when stress becomes distress that you start to feel you can't cope.

THE GOOD, THE BAD AND THE UGLY

Barely a day goes by when we don't read about harmful stress and how it is on the increase. There is always some depressing survey by professor so and so, or research from an American university you've never heard of, that tells you that at least ninety-nine per cent of us are under stress and the remaining one per cent don't know they are stressed. You are warned about the dangers of stress. Stress is bad. Stress can destroy careers, relationships and health. It is the cancer of the twenty-first century. You are urged to calm down or break down.

A few things need to be pointed out here.

First of all, stress is not something new. Longer working days, the lack of job security, commuting, new technology, new choices and the fast pace of modern life all contribute to the increase in stress levels today. But the new millennium didn't invent stress. It has been with us since the beginning of time. What could be more stressful than fighting for survival in prehistoric times, living with disease in the Middle Ages or enduring the horror of a world war? Stress is a fact of life. In times past we endured it, but these days we want to understand it and find ways to minimise it and protect ourselves against it in the future.

Secondly, stress is not an illness. Stress is the result of your response to a situation. It is not something you can catch or something 'out there' waiting to attack that you can do little about.

Thirdly, stress research may not be truly representative. Often the surveys are based on samples of a hundred or so people. But who are these people? What makes them representative? I've never been asked to take part in such a survey. Have you? I'm not saying here that stress isn't a problem for lots of people. It certainly is. What I am saying is that surveys and statistics can sometimes make things seem worse than they are. Not everyone suffering from stress will get ill or depressed. There is every reason to be optimistic that you will be able to overcome stress in your life. Simple, effective methods can reduce stress in the majority of cases. Although we are all under some form of stress, only a tiny percentage of us will actually get seriously ill as a result. You don't have to be one of them.

And finally, what is often overlooked is that stress is essential for human existence. You can't be alive and not experience stress. In moderation stress sharpens your reflexes, heightens your responses and enables you to cope with demanding and difficult situations. If you can learn to use your physical and personal resources to meet the challenge of change, stress can lead to greater self-awareness and self-confidence.

If life was totally stress-free you wouldn't have any difficulties or problems. Life would be predictable. You wouldn't have to adjust to change. You wouldn't ever feel pressured. You, and everyone you know, would be very nice and content. And we'd all be dying of boredom.

One of the most helpful things you can do right now is change your attitude towards stress. Try to think of stress in a more positive light. Stress is the spice of life. In the words of Hans Selye, the doctor who conducted early research into the effects of stress on the body, 'Complete freedom from stress is death because all human activity involves stress.' Stress is a part of life. If you want to avoid it totally, you may as well start looking for a coffin.

The key to a happy, successful life isn't avoiding stress but managing it, and that's what this book is all about. You'll learn how to respond to pressure and how to adapt to change. You'll learn how to take the distress out of stress. You'll learn that you have within you all the resources you need not just to cope with stress, but to thrive on it.

CHAPTER 2

A STATE OF ALERT

If we all knew how to manage stress, stress wouldn't be a problem. Later we'll think about why some of us can cope better with stress than others, but first we need to see how stress affects our bodies and our minds and to be able to identify when stress is harmful and when it isn't.

THE STRESS RESPONSE

When you are under stress your body chemistry changes. The immediate effect of stress-induced tension is a flushed look, increased sweating and a faster or possibly irregular heartbeat. You feel alert and ready for action. You breathe quicker. There may be tingling in the feet and hands. You may feel nauseated, get a butterfly feeling in your stomach and need to use the bathroom. Your hands and feet may feel colder. You could feel faint and weak in the limbs.

All these feelings are caused by your body trying to respond to a physical or emotional stress. Your heart pumps harder and more blood is diverted to the muscles, and so the intestines and other digestive organs receive less. Your mouth feels dry because the glands that produce saliva are part of the digestive system and when they get less blood they are less active. As your muscles receive more blood, they burn up more oxygen from your blood and replace it with carbon dioxide. When carbon dioxide levels rise in your bloodstream, your breathing is stimulated, so you breathe rapidly.

You will also notice all these changes when you feel emotionally tense – angry, anxious, frightened or excited. Your body responds to these emotions and prepares you for action even if that action never arrives. Physical and emotional stress create the same kind of biochemical responses in your body.

These biochemical reactions to stress are healthy and normal. Often described as the flight-or-fight response, they prepare your body for a quick reaction and focus your mind. For instance, you see a vehicle coming and pull your child away from the curb, or you grab the phone to call for help if you hear an intruder in the house. The stress response only becomes harmful when the stress is too intense or continues for too long and the biochemical responses aren't shut off. The body can't return to normal, and stress hormones continue to circulate in the body, doing untold damage.

The body will try to adapt to the stress by releasing more stress hormones to set the body's defences at a higher level. But this can't go on forever, and sooner or later the result is exhaustion. The body, or parts of it, give up the fight.

UNHEALTHY STRESS RESPONSES

Heavy short-term or continuing stress can affect the immune system, making you more prone to infection. Have you noticed that when you are relaxed and happy you don't tend to get as ill as when you are tense and worried? Stress is linked to many commonplace illnesses, such as colds and flu and headaches, as well as more serious conditions such as diabetes, high blood pressure, increased risk of heart attack and cancer.

It has long been known that stress causes indigestion, heartburn and other problems such as irritable bowel syndrome. When you are stressed, a meal that normally doesn't give you problems sends you rushing to the bathroom. The stress reaction closes the digestive system down, shunting blood away from the digestive tract and towards the muscles. Once the blood supply is redirected, food doesn't move along the digestive tract efficiently and digestion is impaired. So even if you are eating a healthy diet, you may not benefit from it if you are under stress.

Stress can also lead to an increase in the production of stomach acid and perhaps even ulcers. If stomach acid is increased, the lining of the digestive tract can be damaged. What's more, if levels of cortisol, a stress hormone, are high, tissue healing in the gut wall is impaired, which can cause leaky gut syndrome. This is when the gut allows tiny pieces of undigested food particles to circulate in the bloodstream. A leaky gut can be a factor in food sensitivities and can result in seemingly unconnected symptoms such as bloating, indigestion, flatulence, constipation, diarrhoea, headaches and rashes.

Stress also interferes with blood sugar levels. The main stress hormone, adrenaline, releases glucose into the bloodstream. Insulin normally steps in afterwards to regulate blood sugars again, but if this happens continuously over long periods it can lead to feeling tired and craving stimulants such as sweets and coffee.

You may find that when you feel tense you feel the urge for foods that can quickly boost your energy. The problem with this quick fix is that it only works as a short-term solution. You get a lift, and that is followed by another dip, which leaves you looking for another fix. It can lead to a vicious circle that causes fatigue, food cravings, weight gain and mood swings. The sugar and refined carbohydrates that fuel blood sugar swings also feed unfriendly gut bacteria, which make gut leakiness worse.

You might think that all that stress would help you lose weight. Wrong. You are more likely to gain it. The effect of stress on body weight differs from person to person. Some people lose weight when they are stressed and gain it when they are happy, but most of us tend to eat for comfort under stress, which increases calorie intake. And even if stress makes you feel less hungry than usual, you may not lose weight. Insulin, which brings blood sugars down, stores excess blood sugar as fat. Your body becomes a fat-friendly machine. You're eating less and weighing more.

So far we've focused on the body rather than the mind, but don't forget that stress can also show itself in abnormal anxiety which destroys quality of life and interferes with quality of sleep. Insomnia is a common symptom of stress. Stress is also linked to mood swings, impulsive, unpredictable behaviour, lack of concentration, low self-esteem and depression.

In short, stress can make you ill, tired and unhappy.

ASSESSING YOUR STRESS LEVELS

In this chapter we've seen how destructive stress can be. Compare too much stress in your life to a car revving endlessly or a washing machine loaded too tightly. Sooner or later something is going to break down. That's why it is important to detect harmful stress sooner rather than later to minimise the damage it can cause.

The way stress affects you depends on a balance between the demands made upon you and your ability to cope with these demands. You need to discover a level of stress that satisfies your need for stimulation and allows you to make adjustment to change smoothly.

Because everyone is unique, only you can know what your stress level is. Think about the level of stress in your life. Is it healthy or harmful? Are you coping with the pressure?

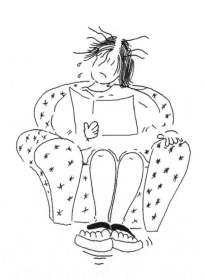

CHAPTER 3

CAN YOU COPE?

Getting stressed is not a sign of weakness. Indeed it is often the case that the strongest, most courageous people are the ones who push themselves to breaking point. Some individuals, though, are more vulnerable to stress than others. Why? Have a think about the following:

- Some studies indicate that the experience gained in childhood and the example set by our caregivers, teachers and peers when dealing with stress is significant. Children are born copycats. They copy what they see, and this could have affected your adult perception of stress and coping with it.

- Some people are more genetically predisposed to stress than others, as they have lower levels of serotonin, a major neurotransmitter having a calming effect. They have a greater tendency to feel anxious and depressed under tension.

- Significant life events can cause stress, such the loss of a loved one, moving to a new house or the birth of a child. Changes, either positive or negative, can up your stress level.

- How much support you get from family, partners, colleagues and friends can make a big difference in your stress responses. Do you have a network of people you can confide in? Feeling connected to the important people in your life can protect you from the more harmful effects of stress. Talking about your fears and anxieties helps bring a sense of relief and perspective.

■ Your gender may also be significant, although this is highly controversial. Professor Shelley Taylor of the University of California, Los Angeles, and senior author of the *Psychological Review*, believes he has discovered a gender difference in the way the sexes respond to stress. According to Taylor's research women are less likely to fly off the handle or bury their feelings when confronted with stress. Men are more likely to respond with aggression or denial. The key to this behaviour difference is the hormone oxytocin, which promotes relaxation and loving feelings. Both men and women produce oxytocin under stress, but women produce more of it.

■ And finally, you need to have a think about your personality. Coming to terms with yourself is the first step on the road to successful stress management Only when you can accept yourself, warts and all, can you start to manage stress successfully. Perfectionists, pessimists and high achievers are more likely to get stressed than those with a hardy personality who are more easygoing, patient and tolerant and able to create a healthy balance in their lives between work, rest and play.

WHAT'S YOUR PROBLEM?

Now that you are working on self-awareness, and better able to identify if you are prone to stress, let's move on to finding out what may be causing you stress. Have a think about the following:

■ not having the right change

- people talking in the cinema
- traffic jams
- the rush hour
- trains running late
- supermarket queues
- the cash machine swallowing your credit card
- not being able to find the can-opener
- not being able to find the corkscrew
- junk mail
- filling in your tax return
- more junk mail
- your computer crashing
- dealing with bureaucracies
- staying in all day for the engineers or delivery men who never arrive
- trying to download from the Internet
- not being able to find a parking spot
- getting an answerphone when you want to speak to a real person and so on.

I don't know about you, but just thinking about the frustration these small irritations cause got my stress levels right up!

It isn't just major life changing events that can cause stress.

What makes stress such a pressing problem today is that there are so many ordinary everyday stressors. Having builders in the house, trying to have sex before your partner falls asleep, trying to get your children into the school of your choice, or simply travelling on the underground can gradually create a build-up of tension and leave you suffering from a wide variety of stress-related symptoms.

NEGATIVE COPING

You may not realise it, but you already have found a way to cope with stress. Unfortunately, the pattern and method you have found may be making stress worse. If you are going to be truly successful in coping with stress, you need to identify negative coping patterns.

Perhaps you are smoking, drinking or taking drugs to calm you. Perhaps you are eating too much or watching too much television. Perhaps you are overspending or engaging in other excessive behaviour. Perhaps emotional outbursts or feelings of helplessness are ways to avoid stress.

Don't feel bad about yourself if you have found unhealthy ways to cope with stress. All I am asking you to do here is identify your pattern of behaviour. Once you become more aware of what you are doing and how you are choosing behaviour that intensifies stress, you can start to replace negative coping patterns with more positive ones.

WORK, REST AND PLAY

Before we move on to stress management strategies, it's important to look at your lifestyle and the way you are coping right now. It is easy to rush off and try stress management techniques, but if you don't think about why you feel the way you do, you are wasting your time. All the pressure is on you to try the latest fad, but in dealing with harmful stress the most important thing is finding out where there is an imbalance in your life.

Forget special diets, yoga retreats and feng shui: finding a balance in your life between work, rest and play is truly the most effective treatment for stress you will find. Does your life look like this? Or more like this?

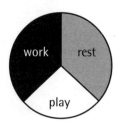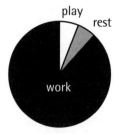

If it looks like the second circle, you need to consider what action you can take to get it more in balance.

Carefully looking at your life may be all that some of you need to reduce stress. You can see where there is an imbalance, and even though it may take time and considerable readjustment, you can get yourself back on track.

It's all too easy today to blame stress for everything. We say stress stops us doing what we want with our lives. There is some truth in this, but let's look at it another way. Maybe the real problem isn't stress. Maybe the real problem is blaming stress for unpleasant feelings and events and then doing nothing about it.

If you are impatient to go on to direct treatments for stress, pause a little and think. Perhaps this attitude is making stress worse. You are suffering from stress, but you aren't addressing the causes. Why not take a long hard look at your life first and see what changes are possible to create more balance in your life between work rest and play. Then, take a deep breath, and come with me to the rest of the book.

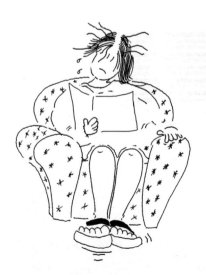

CHAPTER 4

CALMING THE BODY AND MIND

Until your body and mind are calm it's hard to fight stress. You need to feel relaxed before you can start to take a look at your life, identify negative patterns and make positive changes.

THE RELAXATION RESPONSE

Relaxation is the time when you recharge your batteries and focus on what makes you feel good. Under stress you may neglect to set aside time and space for yourself. You may find it hard to relax at all.

When you feel stressed, the muscles in your body tense, and muscular tension creates unpleasant sensations such as headaches, tightness in the chest, difficulty breathing, churning in the stomach, difficulty swallowing. These sensations trigger more tension and a vicious cycle is set up.

You may be able to relax by watching a movie or reading a book or listening to music or playing an instrument, but if you can't relax, you need to learn how. A variety of techniques can be used to achieve this. It doesn't matter which one you choose, the goal is the same – relaxation. You might choose massage, prayer, mediation or yoga. The important thing is to set aside time each day for focused relaxation.

This is a simple way to relax your whole body slowly, muscle by muscle. Start by dropping your shoulders, relaxing the muscles in your body and in your face – it's amazing how many of us frown without knowing it – breathing deeply and gently relaxing. There are many tapes on the market that can help you through the process. You could also try counting to ten before you react, or repeat some positive affirmation to yourself like 'I am in control.'

Try this simple routine. Choose a focus word or phrase – for example, 'peace' or 'happy'. Sit quietly, and relax your body by tensing and then relaxing your muscles and breathing deeply. Say the focus word every time you exhale. If you lose concentration, simply return your thoughts to the word. Try this for just five minutes at first, and then gradually increase the amount of time. Do the routine at least once a day.

Don't expect relaxation to be easy. Relaxing is a skill that has to be practised. You may feel peculiar or uncomfortable at first if you are used to tension. Don't worry about this; just accept that it will take time before you feel comfortable. Make sure that you are breathing deeply and not practising when you are hungry, full or overtired. Make your environment conducive to relaxation. If you get a cramp, ease the tension by rubbing the painful area gently. If you fall asleep easily, you might want to avoid lying down.

CORRECT BREATHING

If you want to relax successfully you need to learn how to breathe properly. A powerful way to produce less stress and more energy in your body is to learn how to breathe with your diaphragm, which literally activates relaxation centres in your brain.

When you are stressed you may hyperventilate or breathe rapidly. This rapid breathing is a natural response to stress or exertion. It uses the upper part of the lungs and results in too much oxygen intake.

Everyone hyperventilates when they are tense or are exercising. We breathe faster to give our muscles oxygen for increased activity to relieve the stress. Rapid breathing isn't a problem if it is short-term, but if it becomes habitual, it results in too much oxygen being taken into the bloodstream. The oxygen-carbon monoxide balance will be upset, causing unpleasant physical symptoms such as tingling in the hands or face, muscle cramps, dizziness, fatigue and aches and pains. These symptoms can be quite alarming and they can trigger another cycle of stress.

It is easy to learn how to breathe correctly when you are anxious. Avoid breathing from your upper chest, and try not to gulp or gasp. When you first try to breathe correctly, you may want to lie down to feel the difference between deep breathing and shallow breathing.

First exhale as much as you can. Then inhale gently and evenly through your nose, filling your lungs completely so that your abdominal muscles move outward. Then exhale slowly and fully. Repeat this, trying to get a rhythm going. You might want to aim to take ten breaths a minute. If you are not getting enough air, return to breathing that is normal for you. Then try increasing the length of one breath, breathing out fully, then in fully, then out again. If that breath felt comfortable, try another one. To get a rhythm going it's important not to try hard but to cooperate as easily as you can with your breathing muscles. Simple yoga breathing exercises – for example, breathing in slowly through the nose while counting to five, holding your breath for a count of five, breathing out slowly through the nose for a count of five, waiting for a count of five and repeating as often as you like – may also help.

It is important to practise correct breathing every time you feel stressed. As you practise you will find that it gets easier and easier to breathe deeply instead of rapidly. Concentrating on breathing and counting can be wonderfully calming for your mind, while the regular breathing will calm the body.

STRESS AND SLEEP

In order to relax successfully you need to feel refreshed and rested. Unfortunately, stress is a great sleep disrupter, resetting your biological clock and causing mental havoc. Under stress, your body is primed for flight or fight, and it takes longer to get to sleep and the quality of your sleep is affected. If you don't get a good night's sleep the quality of your life deteriorates. You feel tired, tense and irritable, your judgment is impaired, it's hard to relax without falling asleep and it's even harder to fight stress.

So what can you do to help you sleep better?

First of all, you need to find out why you aren't sleeping well. It could be that some of the substances you take on a daily basis, such as caffeine and alcohol, are the culprits. The caffeine you drink during the day can remain in your system for up to fifteen hours. So if you are not sleeping well, try to avoid caffeine for ten hours before your bedtime. Have your coffee in the morning if you can, and if you have to drink tea or hot chocolate in the afternoon and evening, make sure they are milky.

Alcohol as a nightcap won't help you either, unless you have just a little, say one or two glasses of wine. Any more than that, and the drinker is likely to wake early after the alcohol has been metabolised and the brain starts to crave more.

Many smokers say that nicotine from cigarettes helps them feel relaxed, but the effect is short-lived. The relaxation is only a result of the craving for nicotine being satisfied. Once the nicotine has been metabolised the brain starts to crave a fresh supply. This disturbs and often wakes up the sleeper. Nicotine patches can help here, because the addict is provided with regular nicotine. We'll look at caffeine, alcohol and smoking in more detail in the next chapter.

Certain medications can also interfere with good quality sleep. Diet pills, for example, often contain caffeine or other stimulants. If you are on any medication, check with your doctor.

Food can be a great sleep disturber, because eating raises your metabolic rate and the body temperature rises, waking you up. Try to avoid large meals in the evening and eating altogether an hour or so before you go to bed. Various food additives have also been linked with sleeping problems; monosodium glutamate and tartrazine (E-102) seem to cause the most trouble. In some circumstances, though, food can be a sleep aid; eating a meal high in fat and low in carbohydrates can make some people feel sleepy. It all depends on the individual. If you suffer from restless legs during the night, extra magnesium might help.

You also need to avoid exercise in the evening. Regular exercise can improve quality of sleep but not if it is done in the evening. Research has shown that even twenty minutes of walking before bedtime can delay sleep by around ten minutes. Take an early morning walk or exercise session instead.

Now that you have pinpointed certain factors that may be interfering with your sleep, you can plan ahead. It sounds strange, but if you are having trouble sleeping you should be preparing for a good night's sleep from the moment you wake up. Exercise in the morning or early afternoon, and have your main meals and most of your caffeine intake in the morning and afternoon as well. As evening approaches, avoid bright light and noise. Bright light in the evening disturbs the biological clock. Make sure curtains close completely and are lined to prevent any light coming through. Temperature is also significant. Body temperature starts to drop at night-time, reaching its lowest point at 4 a.m. Turning down the central heating may help this process; 62°F seems to be most conducive to restful sleep, while higher temperatures can lead to restlessness. Set the timer to come on again at 4 a.m.

By the time you reach bed you should be ready to sleep. You may find that reading makes you feel sleepy, but if you have sleep problems banish all other activities from the bed: no reading, no television, radio, eating or work. If you are still awake after thirty minutes, get up and do something else and don't come back to bed until you are sleepy. If you focus too much on sleep it will elude you, so stop thinking about it. Distract yourself. Read a book, listen to music or try some relaxation techniques.

You may be able to sleep anywhere and comfort may not be a factor. But if it is, consider irregular bed surfaces, smells, dirty bedclothes and soggy mattresses. Mattresses need to be replaced every ten years. Some noise may help you sleep better, such as rhythmic sounds including waves or wind, but heavy noisy will irritate. Once again, it depends on the individual.

Many people find that a relaxing bath helps prepare one for sleep. According to Chinese medicine, baths balance the flow of energy in the body. Research has shown that a warm bath one or two hours before bedtime can help a person sleep better. You might like to get into a routine of bathing every night before you go to bed. For greater relaxation, try adding a chamomile infusion to your bath.

Natural therapies such as massage, yoga, hypnotherapy, reflexology, feng shui, aromatherapy and herbal infusions can all help you sleep better. We'll explore these in more detail later. If you can, avoid sleeping pills. Some doctors believe they are as much a health risk as smoking two packets of cigarettes a day. And sleeping pills create an unnatural sleep state, so when you wake you won't feel so refreshed.

To deal effectively with stress, the art of relaxation is crucial. Once you get used to taking time out and finding ways to calm your body and your mind, you may find that stress simply melts away. If it does, that's great. If, however, you still feel tense and stressed it might be time to start looking at other factors. Don't give up on your relaxation training, though. It's the foundation stone of all stress management techniques.

CHAPTER 5

EATING TO BEAT STRESS

Just when a balanced, wholesome diet is needed most, if you are feeling stressed you may neglect your body's needs. You may have no appetite at all, or you may crave unhealthy and fattening foods. As a result, nutritional deficiencies or imbalances are likely, particularly a lack of B vitamins, folic acid, vitamin C and the minerals calcium, copper, iron, magnesium and potassium.

The relationship between the brain's chemistry and different nutrients is unclear, but nutritional guidelines from the Department of Health offer pointers on nutrition if you suffer from stress. Plenty of wholegrains, peas and lentils and other pulses and regular amounts of lean meat, oily fish, shellfish and eggs will supply B vitamins, iron, potassium, magnesium, copper and zinc. A high intake of fresh fruit and vegetables (such as asparagus, broccoli, cabbage, melon, oranges and berries) will supply ample vitamin C. Dark green leafy vegetables will improve levels of calcium, magnesium and iron, dried fruits will provide potassium and iron, while dairy products (preferably low-fat) will boost levels of calcium. These recommendations can be kept in mind when considering the general guidelines for good diet.

In general, your diet should contain a balanced mix of carbohydrates, proteins and fats. You should be eating enough fibre, ensuring that you get an adequate intake of essential vitamins and minerals and drinking lots of water. Eating to beat stress means concentrating on foods that are not overprocessed and are as fresh and natural in colour as possible. It also means enjoying your food. After all, we're trying to reduce stress here, not add to it, right?

The guidelines given here are in accordance with the Healthy Exchange System originally developed by the American Diabetic Association and other groups for diabetics, but are now used for the design of many therapeutic diets.

Carbohydrate

The World Health Organization (WHO) and the Healthy Exchange System recommend that between fifty and seventy per cent of a person's diet should be carbohydrate. The carbohydrate should come not from foods high in sugar, such as cakes and sweets, but foods rich in complex carbohydrate that offer lasting fuel instead of quick bursts of sugar. Complex carbohydrates are high in fibre, low in starch and sugar, and rich in vitamins and minerals and they help keep blood sugar levels stable. Complex carbohydrate is found in wholegrains, pulses, bread, pasta, rice, potatoes, nuts and seeds, fruits and vegetables and salads.

Best high-quality carbohydrate: Fruits – apples, oranges, grapefruit, strawberries, pears, peaches and plums. Vegetables – broccoli, asparagus, green beans, cauliflower and spinach. Grains – barley, rye, brown rice, wholemeal bread and pasta. Beans – black beans, white beans, chickpeas, kidney beans and lentils.

You should have five servings of fruit, vegetables or salad a day and four servings of carbohydrate, from other sources. A serving is one medium-sized apple and one medium slice of bread.

Protein

Protein should make up around fifteen per cent of your diet. Protein is found in meat, dairy produce, eggs, fish, poultry, pulses, nuts and seeds. Try to choose proteins that are low in saturated fats. Proteins are the essential building blocks of cells and a healthy nervous system; fish, lean poultry, pulses and soya are some of the best sources. You should aim to have two servings a day of non-dairy products and one serving a day of a dairy product. A serving is two ounces of cheese or one egg.

Fat

Fats should make up around twenty to twenty-five per cent of your diet. Fats are found in most foods. Too much of the wrong sort of fat is bad for you. Avoid saturated fats from animal products and fats that are solid at room temperature, such as lard and butter. Fats that are liquid at room temperature, such as vegetable oils, are far preferable, since they don't contain the chemicals that can clog arteries.

It is important to ensure an adequate intake of essential fats, which build healthy cell membranes and nervous tissue and balance hormones. The best sources are oily fish, fresh nuts, fresh seeds and cold-pressed oils such as olive, flax, walnut, sesame and sunflower.

Fibre

An adequate intake of dietary fibre is also important. WHO recommends around 30 g of fibre a day. Food high in fibre include fruits and vegetables, brown bread, rice and pasta, high fibre cereals, potatoes and baked beans. A jacket potato contains around 5 to 8 g per serving.

Fibre swells the bulk of the food residue in the intestine and helps to soften it by increasing the amount of water retained. It is vital to the health of the digestive system, and many ailments, such as irritable bowel, constipation and piles, result if you don't get enough. Western diets are often low in fibre, and those who eat a lot of processed and refined food are vulnerable. But there are easy ways to boost fibre intake:

- Have a bowl of high-fibre cereal for breakfast

- Eat brown bread, pasta and rice

- Snack on fruits and nuts rather than crisps and chocolate.

High-fibre foods are nutritious and can satisfy without being fattening. Some types of fibre – those found in vegetables, fruits and oats – can reduce blood cholesterol. Cholesterol is a variety of fat that has some health benefits, so it shouldn't be excluded from a diet, but too much cholesterol is linked to clogging of the arteries, especially those around the heart.

Water
Water makes up around seventy per cent of your body, and staying hydrated helps to keep you healthy. Coffee, tea and alcohol are all dehydrating and don't count towards your liquid intake.

The chances are you are not drinking enough water. Ideally, you should be drinking at least six to eight glasses of water a day to maintain health and flush toxins out of the body. For variety, mix sparkling water with some juice. Try a cup of hot water with the juice of lemon or some honey.

Drink a glass of water when you feel hungry; you could be mistaking thirst signals for hunger. Even if you are not, water prepares your digestive system before you eat.

How much should I be eating?

If you follow the basic serving guidelines given above, you should be eating a diet that is high in nutrients and sensible in calories. Calorie counting as a means of determining the healthful nature of your diet rarely works, because when you focus on calories you often neglect the importance of getting all your nutrients. A diet high in essential nutrients is far more effective in combating anxiety and stress than a calorie-controlled diet. You may find that a nutritious diet helps you lose weight more effectively too.

So forget calorie counting, and focus on nutrients.

How often should I be eating?

It seems that eating smaller, more frequent meals rather than larger, fewer ones will help reduce stress levels. Eating breakfast like a king, lunch like a prince and dinner like a pauper can improve alertness and a sense of well-being.

Breakfast is the most important meal of the day, and ideally it should be the largest. Healthy breakfast choices include wholegrain cereals, muffins and breads along with fresh fruit, cereals, lean meat, cheese, yoghurt or eggs. The complex carbohydrates give you the energy boost you need at the start of the day.

A light snack of fruit, vegetable, nuts or seeds around mid-morning will keep your energy levels high. Lunch is a good time to enjoy a nourishing bowl of soup or salad along with some wholegrain bread, lean meat, fish, egg or cheese. This may be followed by another light snack around tea time.

Dinner should be the smallest meal of the day and preferably eaten more than two hours before going to bed. Wholegrains and legumes can be eaten in salads, main dishes and soups. It really doesn't make sense to eat a large meal when you are not going to need much energy. Give your body the time to rest, cleanse and recharge itself for the next day.

Food intolerances

If you suffer from stress, you may need to consider the possibility of intolerance to certain foods, also known as food allergies or sensitivities. As far back as 1930 Dr Albert Row noted that anxiety and fatigue were key features of certain food sensitivities. Other health problems linked to food allergies include depression, inability to concentrate and irritability. Food allergies can become addictive and you may start to crave the very foods to which you are sensitive. It's a hard habit to break.

Possible symptoms of food allergies include bloating, headaches, sluggish metabolism, skin and bowel problems, and mysterious aches and pains. If you think you have a food allergy, it might be worth avoiding the food you suspect for a fortnight to see if you feel any better. This is called the 'food challenge' method of diagnosis. Laboratory methods are also available, such as blood tests, which can provide immediate identification of suspected allergies but are expensive.

Once the food allergy is detected, the best approach is to deal with it through avoidance. The most common food intolerances are to wheat, dairy produce, nuts, eggs, yeast, shellfish, citrus fruits and artificial colourings. Food allergy, to wheat gluten especially, has been linked to depression.

If you are sensitive to wheat, try:

- Rye: ryvita, rye bread, rye slims
- Oats: porridge, oatcakes, flapjacks
- Rice: rice cereals, rice cakes
- Buckwheat
- Quinoa, millet, barley.

If you are sensitive to cow's milk products, try:

- Rice milk, oat milk, yoghurts
- Soya milk, soya yoghurt, soya cheese, tofu
- Coconut milk, almond milk
- Goat's milk, goat's cheese
- Ewe's milk, Ewe's cheese.

Daylight

One final word on nutrients: one of your most important sources has nothing to do with the foods you eat. That source is sunlight. Sunlight supplies vitamin D and it is easy to become deficient if you stay indoors too much. A simple way to deal with this is to go outside and get fresh air as much as you can. Even if it is cold outside and the sun isn't out, the light is good for you and will make you feel better. Don't take this to extremes, though. Too much sun can damage your skin. Once again, moderation is key.

Breaking bad habits

The healthy diet guidelines will improve digestive function, and if you have leaky gut symptoms, a healthy diet will tone the gut and help it heal. It is crucial at this stage that you start to eliminate unhealthy food choices.

Just as important, if not more so, is eliminating addictive stimulants. The trouble with these stimulants, which give temporary energy boosts, is that in the long term they add to your body's stress. As we look at the most common harmful addictions below, try not to think in terms of denying yourself. Where possible, I have suggested healthy options and alternatives.

To find out how much of an impact various substances have upon you, try going without for a few days. You may experience headaches, spots, cloudy urine and unpleasant breath at first, but after a day or two you will get a feeling of lightness and energy as your body is freed from the burden of coping with toxins.

SMOKING

If you think that smoking helps you cope with stress, you couldn't be more wrong. Smoking places a tremendous amount of stress on your body in every way. There are thousands of chemicals in cigarette smoke, apart from the damage caused by nicotine and tar. The toxins in the smoke can interfere with the work of important vitamins and minerals. It uses up vitamin C, which is needed to help ward off illness and keep your skin looking smooth and fresh. That's why smokers tend to be more susceptible to colds and flu and their skin has a dry, wrinkled look.

If you have smoked for years, the last thing you probably want to hear in a book about stress management is advice to give up. This is bound to increase your stress levels one hundred per cent. Without cigarettes, you fear you will put on weight, become irritable and depressed and so on. There's no easy way to say this, so I may as well be direct: If you are serious about reducing stress levels in your life, giving up smoking has to be a priority.

It might help to consider all the benefits of being a non-smoker:

- saving money
- breathing easier
- having fresh breath
- enjoying the taste of food
- losing that smoker's cough
- fewer chest infections
- avoiding smoking-related illness
- fewer wrinkles
- improving the health of your family
- generally feeling happier, healthier and more energetic.

To give up smoking, try to avoid situations and people that you associate with smoking, for example, the pub. If you always have a cigarette first thing in the morning, brush your teeth or read a paper instead. Pick a stop day, preferably at the weekend when you are less stressed, and start to cut down a few weeks beforehand. The day before you give up, throw away ashtrays and lighters. Have your last cigarette and the next day start your day in a different way.

Change your routines to avoid situations when you might feel tempted, keep yourself busy and constantly remind yourself of the long-term benefits. For every day that you don't smoke, give yourself a huge pat on the back. You need to be prepared for withdrawal symptoms and cravings. There may also be mood swings and a cough when your lungs clear. You can use nicotine patches or gum, but in the long run they really aren't that helpful as they can be addictive as well. There may be a slight weight gain due to a decrease in your metabolic weight and an increased food intake, but you can get this under control by concentrating on the healthy diet guidelines given above.

Caffeine

Sources of caffeine include coffee, tea, chocolate, colas, energy drinks, headache medication and painkillers. Caffeine can reduce your ability to cope under pressure. It overstimulates the adrenal glands, which seems to help in the short term but makes matters worse in the long term. Even moderate doses of caffeine can raise levels of stress hormones, adrenaline and cortisol, to higher levels than those normally produced by the stress response. Caffeine can also interfere with the absorption of important stress-busting nutrients such as zinc and B vitamins.

You don't need to cut out caffeine entirely; you just need to take it in moderation. One or two cups of coffee a day for instance, not ten. You may find barley, chicory or dandelion good substitutes for coffee. Green tea, red bush tea, ginger tea, fruit tea or hot cordial can be good tea substitutes. As for chocolate, try dried fruit bars or fruit and grain bars, dried fruit mixed with fresh nuts or a low-sugar cereal bar or seventy per cent cocoa solid chocolate bar as alternatives. Herbal drinks or juice mixed with sparkling water can be enjoyable.

Alcohol

Like caffeine, alcohol overstimulates the adrenal glands, but this time the effect on blood sugar levels and brain chemistry is more significant. Alcohol depletes the body of essential vitamins and minerals. Alcohol also triggers the need to snack more, and drinking too much provides empty calories, which contribute to weight gain. You don't need to stop drinking entirely; you just need to cut down to sensible amounts. In fact, four measures a week of alcohol can be quite good for you. The rest of the time try sparkling water, fruit juice, herbal drinks like Aqua Libra, or mix your wine with sparkling water.

Sugar and salt

Refined white sugar also sends your blood-sugar levels up, affects your mood and makes you gain weight, in addition to rotting your teeth. It also impairs the working of the adrenal glands and suppresses the immune system. Many of the foods, especially processed foods, we eat today are packed with hidden sugars and most of us consume far too much.

If you have a sweet tooth, you might want to try eating fruit rather than sweets, biscuits and cakes. Read the package labels of the food you buy and try fructose sugar from health food shops, which does not unbalance blood sugar, or fructo-oligosaccharides, a sweet-tasting powder. Try adding honey or fruit to cereals and desserts, and eat more wholegrains and fruits to reduce your dependency on sugar. Sweeteners aren't really a good idea because they don't retrain your sweet tooth.

Moderation in salt is also advised. Excessive intake of salt can promote fluid retention and cause a rise in blood pressure, and an increased risk of stroke, heart disease and kidney failure. Much processed food contains salt. Crisps are high in salt, and lots of us sprinkle salt on our food, which isn't necessary.

One final word about cravings: the next time you crave something stop and think what you are actually wanting. Remind yourself that you don't have to have anything just because you desire it. You are in control. Also remember that one lapse isn't the end of the world. We all have good or bad days. Just pick yourself up and start again – it's that simple. Avoiding difficult situations until you feel in control may also help, such as not filling the fridge with unhealthy food. And remember, it will take time. Some days it will be harder than others. But if you keep working at it, in time you will be able to replace old habits with new healthier ones.

In this chapter we've looked at two of the most helpful ways you can stress-proof your life. Simple adjustments in your diet, as well as eliminating toxic stimulants, can make a huge difference. Let's now take a look at another vital component of a comprehensive stress management programme and overall good health: exercise.

CHAPTER 6

KEEPING FIT

Every time we suffer from harmful stress, we put our bodies and minds temporarily out of balance. The fitter we are the more rapidly we return to normal. An overweight person with furred-up arteries has so little in reserve that even a minor stress, such as climbing a few stairs, can prove too demanding – with fatal consequences.

Exercise is more than just a way to sweat calories and lose weight. It has a powerful effect on your mind and your body, counteracting the effect of pent-up tension from inactivity and boosting levels of beta-endorphins, the naturally occurring opiates that lift our mood. Other nerve chemicals such as adrenaline, serotonin and dopamine are also secreted in the brain during exercise. Exercise can help reduce anxiety and depression and stimulate a feeling of well-being.

There is no one best way to keep fit. Your choice of exercise will depend on your personality. The important thing is that it involves your whole body, increases your heart rate and makes you a little breathless. Even if a short lunchtime stroll is all you can manage, you can still expect physical and mental gains. Research has shown that a short ten-minute walk can leave subjects feeling relaxed and energetic. Other studies compare exercise benefits to the benefits gained from a course of psychotherapy. It improves body image, builds self-esteem and helps you cope with stress.

But what about those of us who really don't like exercise or simply have not got the time? The answer is to find a form of exercise you enjoy. If you dread your workouts, stop them and do something different. Perhaps you would feel more committed to exercise if you found an activity that was social and included other people, such as dancing or exercise classes. If you hate gyms, try to incorporate toning and strengthening exercises into your daily life. For example, you can tighten your buttocks while you sit at your desk, or try to improve your posture. Make your daily life a little more active. Putting more energy into everyday chores such as housework or gardening can burn calories and build muscle tone too.

Many people who hate exercise actually find that they enjoy walking. Walking really doesn't seem like exercise, but the benefits of a regular walking programme are incredible. You can walk indoors or outdoors. Try to start including it into your daily schedule and if possible, it may even become your means of transport. Make sure you don't carry heavy bags when you walk and that you wear supportive walking shoes. Aim for a pace that makes your heart beat a little faster, and if fat burning is your goal, try to walk at least five times a week. You can walk every day as long as you don't push yourself. The question of how often you can walk is less important than how long you walk. If your schedule is too tight for long walks, there are still benefits to several short walks every day. Even a few minutes of exercise a day are beneficial.

Always warm up before you do any sort of exercise, however short. And remember that muscles need stretching before and after strengthening.

POSTURE

Suffering from stress can affect our posture. Good posture is critical to our well-being. It makes us look and feel taller, thinner, more energetic and more sure of ourselves.

There are ways you can improve your posture. First of all, you need to become aware that the muscles of alignment are situated at the back of our body not the front. That is why sucking in our tummies or pulling back our shoulders will just tire us out instead of improving our shape. The muscles at the front of the body are not meant to be stabilising, but the muscles that run along the back and spine and legs are. As we are not used to using these muscles at first, they may need retraining. This may explain why you may find it hard to stand balanced on both feet rather than shifting from one to the other, or to sit with legs uncrossed rather than crossed.

Fortunately, once you start thinking of the back-to-front way to use your muscles, it won't take long to adjust; the stomach naturally flattens and your shape improves.

To do a quick check on your posture, have a look at yourself sideways in a mirror. Let your tailbone point downward toward the floor. Rather than sticking out your chest, let your collarbones gently reach for the sky. Release all tension in your shoulders and neck and feel as if someone is pulling you from the centre of your head with a string. If you look at yourself now, you will realise how slumped you normally are. You'll also see how good posture can take kilos off you and make you look more confident and poised.

Body mechanics are also important to avoid stress and

tension. When bending or lifting, plant the feet firmly apart and bend the knees so that the back stays straight and long. Hold an object you are lifting close to you, and lift it by straightening your knees, not your back. Lift upward when you sit, too, and try to avoid crossing your legs. This can be a hard habit to break, but if continued it will really weaken the lower back muscles. Work at desks that are the right height for you and that help you keep your back long. When driving, make sure your knees are slightly higher than your hips. And if you must wear high heels, wear them for short periods only. High heels shift the centre of gravity forward and distort your posture and put the body under tremendous strain.

WEIGHT MANAGEMENT

One of the most unpleasant side-effects of stress is weight gain. The theory is that stress hormones affect the type of fat that settles beneath the abdominal wall. Basically stress increases your waistline and accelerates weight gain.

There are hundreds of programmes to help you manage your weight. Some promise miracle results in a short period of time. Each of them has a different approach. The truth, though, is that no one solution will work for everyone. A method of weight loss that works for you won't work for someone else. You have to find what suits you. But if you want to lose weight, four diet rules will always apply:

1. Lose weight gradually. Statistics prove that drastic weight loss is seldom effective and is usually dangerous. Aim for a loss of about half a kilo a week. A good weight-loss programme

ensures that you lose weight gradually and do not see it go on again when you stop.

2. Increase your activity levels. Basically, move about more. A regular programme of exercise that includes aerobic, strengthening and stretching exercise is best if you can manage it. If you lose weight by diet alone, you will just look flabby and out of shape. Exercise gives you shape and tone. It helps flatten your stomach and waist and your hips to look firmer. Exercise burns calories, but what is more important is that you build up muscle mass through exercise. Muscles burn calories more efficiently than fat. The more lean muscle tissue you have, the higher your metabolism will be. The higher your metabolism, the faster you will lose weight and burn up fat stores.

   An exercise programme for weight loss should include at least forty-five minutes of aerobic exercise at least four times a week. To burn fat you also need to build up your muscle strength. Muscles need more energy than fat and burn up calories faster. Strength training needs to be a part of a weight-loss programme, and don't forget the importance of stretching and lengthening your body every time you start and finish your exercise routine.

3. Eat to lose weight. You need a balance of all the essential nutrients to feel healthy and to lose weight. Refer back to Chapter 5 for healthy and fun guidelines for getting all the essential nutrients. Losing weight safely and effectively is a matter of eating food that can boost our metabolism and burning up more energy than we use from our food. Foods rich in nutrients have magic properties that can eliminate hunger,

erase water weight and speed up your body's fat-burning power. The more nutrient-rich foods you eat, the slimmer you can get. You won't feel hungry all the time, either. Remember to drink lots of water also, to keep your tissues well lubricated and to help flush out water weight.

Some foods can interfere with metabolism and make you feel bloated and heavy. These include synthetic food additives, processed foods, foods high in salt, coffee, chocolate and foods high in saturated fat and sugar. Try always to eat quality, wholesome foods free of additives and rich in nutrients. Avoid fast food which is refined or processed or packed with sodium and synthetic additives. These kinds of foods don't have the substances you need for weight loss. Concentrate on whole, unrefined and fresh foods rich in nutrients.

4. Change your eating habits for life. In order to lose weight permanently you need to change your eating habits for the rest of your life. More fruits and vegetables, less fat and sugar, reduction in servings and an adequate intake of nutrients are the best and most effective ways to lose weight.

Time and time again people go on diets to lose weight and then put it all back on again. If you want to lose weight and keep it off, it is important not to go back to old eating habits. If you do, weight will pile back on again. Instead of dieting, think more of a permanent change in eating habits. From now on you are going to eat to maximise your chances not only of permanent weight loss, but of good health and vitality as well.

In this chapter we've looked at ways stress can be reduced by regular exercise and sensible weight management. Keeping fit trains your body to protect you from future stress and helps you cope with current stress. Along with diet, it is a great way to help yourself to a new, vibrant lease on life. But it isn't just your body you should be training, as the next chapter will show; you need to train your mind as well.

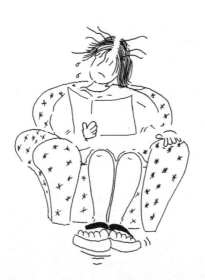

CHAPTER 7

THINKING ERRORS

When you feel stressed you tend to have worrying thoughts. These thoughts or images make you feel anxious and uncertain. It's often the case that unhelpful thinking has become so habitual that you aren't even aware you are doing it. The problem is that the more negative your thoughts, the more negative you are likely to feel, and this can stop you taking positive action to relieve stress.

The first thing you need to do is to become aware of unhelpful thinking patterns. Once you are able to recognise them, you may be able to reduce the problem. Psychologists refer to unhelpful thinking patterns as 'thinking errors'. Under stress, you may find yourself making thinking errors, such as: thinking in all or nothing terms – one mistake and you are a failure; seeing only the negative in a situation; blaming yourself for everything; losing perspective and blowing things out of proportion – it isn't a mistake it is a DISASTER; telling yourself you just can't cope any more and so on.

Becoming aware of how your thoughts are affecting your feelings can be a big step forward. The next time you are stressed, pay attention to your thought processes, and ask yourself which thinking errors you are making. Once you start to recognise negative thought patterns, you can start to replace them with more realistic thoughts. This will also help you distance yourself from stress-inducing thoughts. Changing your thoughts can change your life, which is the basis of a kind of treatment called cognitive therapy.

You may argue that this just isn't realistic. You'd like to be more positive, but sometimes negative thoughts and outcomes are accurate. This may have a grain of truth in it. It's unrealistic to expect positive outcomes to everything. You set yourself up for disappointment.

But psychologists and psychiatrists have shown that under stress people are often biased towards anything that is negative. They also don't always get their facts right. Negative thinkers don't often question the accuracy of their thoughts. They tend to believe that what they think is the truth, but on many occasions it simply isn't. The next time you are negative about something, ask yourself if you are seeing all sides of the picture. Try to distinguish between a negative view that is realistic and a negative view that is misleading or doesn't take into account other possibilities.

Don't always believe everything you think. Question it.

You don't always believe the things other people tell you or what you read in the papers, so why accept everything your thoughts tell you? It's incredible how many inaccuracies are revealed when you start challenging negative thinking.

You don't have to replace negative thoughts with positive ones, simply more appropriate ones. Positive thinking can be as unhelpful and as unrealistic as negative thinking. Always looking on the bright side when things are clearly falling apart around you won't do you any good at all.

Negative thoughts need to replaced with more realistic ones, but fortunately realistic thoughts are much more optimistic than negative ones. Realistic thoughts take into account the negative, but they also take into account the positive. For example, saying to yourself, 'They didn't want me for the job, I'll never get another job', can be replaced by, 'I could get the job, but if I'm not right for it there are other jobs I can apply for.'

When negative thoughts start to appear, evaluate them carefully. Don't treat them automatically as facts because you are thinking them. Most of the time they are inaccurate, misleading and unrealistic. Every time you get a negative, worrying thought, try to challenge it rationally and replace it with more realistic thoughts. The trick is to recognise when you have a worrying thought and to ask yourself, 'Am I being realistic?' If you aren't being realistic, you need to replace the thought with something more constructive.

Research has shown that challenging negative thinking can help reduce stress. Acquiring new thinking skills is the same as learning any new skill: you need to work hard and practise, practise, practise. Now you have identified the common thinking errors that may apply to you, here are some ways to start challenging them:

IT'S A SET-BACK, NOT A FAILURE

If there is a person alive who never make a mistake, I don't think I would like to meet that person. She or he must be very boring indeed.

Everyone makes mistakes. In fact, the most interesting, exceptional people are the ones who make the most. The only way to learn about your strengths and your weaknesses is to make mistakes. Making mistakes builds character.

Negative thinking can really handicap you when you are trying to achieve a new goal or solve a problem. Every mistake you make will be interpreted as a failure and proof of your inadequacy. Of course failures can be devastating, but they can also help you grow and learn about yourself and what you do and do not want in life. You can gain something from every experience, however disappointing. In that light, there is no such thing as a failure.

Rather than labelling your mistakes as failures, try to view them as set-backs or learning experiences. This is less final than failure. Think in terms of temporary set-backs, which add to your store of knowledge whenever you feel disappointed or let down. That way you will feel less inclined to give up and more willing to try again.

Everywhere you turn there are examples of set-backs leading to success. Barbara Streisand, John Grisham, Elvis Presley are just a few examples of people whose ideas were initially rejected but who eventually achieved spectacular success. Sometimes when you are tuning in to a radio station you get the wrong wavelength. You keep fiddling with the tuner until you get the quality of reception that you want. Persistent effort pays off. Just because you didn't get the radio station the first time doesn't mean that you will never get it.

If you are prone to generalisation and sweeping conclusions whenever you have a set-back, you need to start challenging your thought patterns. Fallibility is part of being human. Don't let yesterday's or today's disappointments stop you from succeeding tomorrow. Nobody knows what the future holds. Just because you had a set-back doesn't mean things won't work out another time.

COMPROMISE

All-or-nothing thinking sets you up for disappointment and heartache. It is impossible to do something perfectly, especially if you have made only a few attempts at it. There will always be room for improvement, however brilliant you are.

You may think, 'What's the point, if I'm never going to be one hundred per cent right or the best at what I do?' The point is that there are a lot of advantages to learning new skills. Many great rewards are gained by getting better and better at something. Also, just because you aren't perfect at something doesn't mean that you can't do it well and get lots of satisfaction from it.

If you catch yourself thinking in all-or-nothing terms, try to challenge this by seeing the advantages in your situation. Don't overlook degree or compromise. Tell yourself, 'I didn't get it quite right, but I am getting better all the time.'

It can be helpful to replace shoulds, musts and oughts with less emotionally charged expressions. Use words like 'I could', it is 'preferable' or 'desirable'. And try not to blow the negative components of a situation out of all proportion. A late train isn't the end of the world. When we elevate our response to a situation, we create more stress and minor set-backs can become nightmares.

IT'S NOT ALWAYS YOUR FAULT

Humankind is always trying to explain why things happen. If things don't work out we want to find someone to blame. We blame others. Under stress we tend to blame ourselves.

It's often the case when a natural disaster or a terrible accident occurs that a number of things have contributed. It can be hard to point the finger of blame at just one thing. It's the same for our personal lives. When something goes wrong there are usually a number of reasons why. Some of these things may have been out of our control.

If you have a tendency to blame yourself when things go wrong, closely examine the circumstances that led to the setback. Some of these may have had nothing to do with you.

If you feel you didn't make a good impression when you met a new group of people, try to think why. Maybe you weren't feeling well or were tired. Perhaps the people you met were not very supportive. Perhaps you didn't have much in common with them. None of this is your fault.

Don't try to accept blame for things that are out of your control. Don't concentrate solely on your weaknesses, forgetting the positive aspects and signs of your strengths. When things go wrong, get out of the habit of saying it's your fault because you aren't good enough. Even if you do make mistakes, this doesn't make you worthless. Try to replace blaming thoughts with encouraging ones: 'This didn't work out, but how was I to know this or that would happen?'

It is impossible for you to be in control of all the factors that create a situation. If a friend or colleague made a similar mistake would you be as harsh with them? Probably not. Many of us are supportive of others but overcritical of ourselves. Instead of blaming yourself and seeing only what is wrong, step back and recognise what you did well and what needs your attention.

YOU DON'T KNOW WHAT IS GOING TO HAPPEN

Some things are likely to happen. The sun will rise in the morning and set in the evening. At night the moon and stars will come out.

But there is no such thing as complete certainty. The world probably won't, but it could, end tomorrow!

When you get stressed and start to see only the negative, you lose a sense of perspective. You also forget that you are only human. You can't see into the future. How do you know that things are going to go horribly wrong?

It's more realistic to think that unpleasant things may or may not happen. It's more appropriate to conclude that someone is likely to think in a certain way, but you are not a mind reader. Things may turn out bad, but they may also turn out well. Start allowing yourself the possibility that things may go right. Get rid of over-the-top pessimism.

FINDING AN ALTERNATIVE WAY TO THINK

Negative thinking can be very discouraging and you will often feel like giving up. But if you can challenge negative thoughts by looking for facts to disprove them, you will start to learn that negative thinking not only makes you feel stressed and unhappy, it is also misleading and inaccurate.

Finding an alternative way to think is not the same as positive thinking. Rather, it is about keeping your thoughts in perspective and being realistic. And remember, thinking new thoughts is like any new skill: it takes time, work, and practice. You may not be responsible for the causes of stress in your life, but if you can start to recognise and challenge your thinking errors it may be possible to reduce the amount of distress they cause you.

CHAPTER 8

STRESS MANAGEMENT SECRETS

In this chapter and the next you'll learn additional stress management techniques. All of them are effective in reducing stress and improving the quality of your life. Let's start with time management.

TIME MANAGEMENT

Under stress many of us become efficient procrastinators. If you are one of those people who finds all sorts of unnecessary things to do when deadlines approach or decisions need to be made, and you convince yourself that you work best when everything is last-minute, time management is an important skill for you to learn.

Adding structure to your life can reduce time spent each day getting stressed about what you have forgotten, what you should be doing and where things are. For example, if you are worried about being late, plan your journey and allow yourself enough time. If you worry about losing your keys, have one place where you put them.

You can avoid a lot of stress simply by being more organised. Try to plan ahead as much as you can, put your clothes out the night before, prepare that speech in time, write a shopping list before you go to the supermarket so you don't forget things you need and so on. Writing a daily schedule will also help.

Time management is straightforward, but you will need to make certain changes and learn some new skills. Before you reorganise yourself you need to look at your present routine, what your priorities are and what your goals are.

Organise your day. There will always be unplanned demands on your time, but try to create a definite plan for your day based on your priorities. Tackle the hardest jobs first when you have the most energy. Avoid putting things off until the last minute. You may find that you need to delegate some of your tasks. It's hard to do everything yourself.

In order to manage your time effectively you need to devise a system that meets your needs but that is also flexible. If you think you haven't got time to sit down and think about your schedule, remind yourself that time management is an investment that will pay off. You will feel calmer, better prepared, and more in control of your life.

PROBLEM SOLVING

Indecision can be a major cause of stress. Not knowing what to do about a particular situation or problem simply increases the stress. If you find yourself stuck in worry, uncertainty and indecision, the problem-solving approach may help. Taking action when faced with problems can be far less stressful than feeling anxious about them.

There are several stages in decision making and problem solving. First of all, find out what is making you stressed and see if you can do something about it. Try to solve only the problems you have a chance of solving.

The second stage is listing as many ways as you can of dealing with the cause of your stress, also called brainstorming. At this stage you need to give yourself as much choice as possible. The more choice you have, the more chance you have of selecting a way of coping that is right for you. List as many solutions as you can even if they seem far-fetched. Suspend your judgment and all the reasons why this or that isn't a good solution, and let those ideas come.

When you've listed as many solutions as you can, even the trivial and outrageous ones, now it's time to make a decision.

Get a pen and paper and write down all the positives and negatives linked with the choice you want to make. This will help give you a balanced view of the situation and what kind of consequences to expect. For instance, if you can't make up your mind whether to get married or not, the advantage would be that you take your relationship to a level of deeper commitment. The disadvantage would be that you or your partner might feel a certain loss of freedom.

When weighing up the pros and cons you need to think about what you really want. Sometimes our real needs aren't readily apparent. You may think you want something but you may also feel that you have to act as others expect you to act. Have a think about how many of your ideas and values are yours and reflect who you really are. It is vital that you make a choice which is your choice and reflects what you think is best, not what others expect of you.

When you consider your options, think carefully if this is what you want. Or is it what your mother, your friend, your partner or your colleagues want. For instance, do you really want to get married right now? If you always think 'I should do this', or 'I should do that', start thinking about 'I want to do this', instead, or better still, 'This is in everybody's better interests, including my own'.

Once you start to think about what you really want, life gets a lot easier. You start doing what is right for you and not what others think is right for you. You start considering options and making choices you may not have considered before. You become your own person. And that's when life really gets exciting.'

Earlier I suggested that when you think of solutions to a problem you list as many choices as you can, even ones that seem impossible or unrealistic. This process helps you think up as many solutions as possible and stops you thinking that there isn't an answer. However, once you have thought of a number of coping strategies, it is time to use your common sense. Don't try to solve a problem in a way that isn't suited to your abilities. We all have limitations. Problems often test our limitations.

If you set unrealistic goals, you set yourself up for stress and unhappiness. Sometimes in a strange way failure is reassuring. It makes the world less unpredictable, and if you know you are going to fail you can use your incompetence or hopelessness as an excuse or a way of getting other people to solve a problem for you. So be careful. Don't try to solve a problem that needs skills you don't have or can't acquire. Ask for help if you need it.

If you keep approaching a problem in a way that has failed for you in the past, then try to change your approach and think about whether the solution you are choosing suits with the demands of the coping strategy you have selected.

In very specific and concrete ways, decide what will be done, how it will be done, when it will be done, where it will be done, who is involved and what your backup plan is if something goes wrong. For instance, you may decide that you do really want to change jobs and that you are going to apply for this new one. You decide not to tell your employer unless you get the job. If possible, rehearse in role play or imagination your chosen solution. Now you are ready to move to the final stage: putting your solution into action.

Make sure you are well prepared, and then try out your solution. Whether or not the solution is successful, review it and see what you can learn from the experience.

If your solution worked, congratulate yourself. You may, for example, be offered the job of your dreams. You might like to treat yourself. If you aren't used to treating yourself, think about something you would like and indulge yourself. The important thing is to acknowledge your successes. Also, make time to think about why your solution worked and what you can learn about your strengths and weaknesses from it.

If your solution didn't work, don't torture yourself with self-doubt or anxiety. Try to understand why it didn't work. Say you didn't get offered the job you wanted. Perhaps you just didn't have enough experience. Perhaps you didn't take something into account. Perhaps you weren't feeling strong that day, perhaps you misinterpreted something, perhaps you didn't have a backup plan or were not prepared enough.

Whatever conclusion you reach, remind yourself that you have not failed. Congratulate yourself for having the courage to try. Learn as much as you can from the experience and with the knowledge that you have gained, select another solution and try again. The more solutions you try, the more you will learn and the better equipped you will be to deal with the situation.

Personal success is not about banishing all stress, uncertainty and disappointment. A huge part of mastering personal success is learning how to cope with negative feelings and experiences. It is about experiencing the good and the bad. Mistakes, set-backs and disappointments are part of life and an important part of how we learn and grow. The main difference between those who succeed in life and those who don't is that those who succeed learn from their mistakes.

MORE STRESS MANAGEMENT SECRETS

So far we've seen how time management and problem solving can minimise stress. It's now time to discuss self-awareness, improving your communication skills and emotional confidence.

BE YOURSELF

Self-esteem is a word often used today. Basically it means feeling good about yourself and your life. However confident you are, there are going to be times in everyone's life when self-esteem plummets and during these times you are more vulnerable to stress.

When self-esteem is low you may feel inferior to others and doubt yourself and your abilities. You have problems communicating your needs, feelings and rights to others. You don't feel that you can ask for what you want. It's hard for you to say no without feeling guilty. You don't recognise that it is okay to have opinions, make mistakes, make decisions, be successful, be unsuccessful, change your mind, be independent or need personal space. Other people walk all over you because you find it hard to stand up for yourself. You put the needs of others above your own, and this can cause resentment.

Or low self-esteem could manifest itself in a display of arrogance and false confidence. You feel threatened by other people, rarely listen to them and feel valued only when you are being forceful and can get your way. Or your self-esteem could be so fragile that it depends on externals like your job, your relationship, your weight.

If you are to manage stress successfully, protecting yourself against low self-esteem is crucial. Part of the problem, however, may be in your understanding of the term itself. To avoid confusion, instead of self-esteem I'll use the term self-awareness.

Self-awareness starts by acknowledging that we are all fallible human beings capable of making mistakes. When we are self-aware, our confidence is based not on the way we look, or the job or car we have, but on accepting ourselves warts and all. When you become self-aware you understand and accept yourself. This doesn't meant you don't try to change for the better; it just means that you don't pressure yourself to be perfect.

When you start to accept yourself you start to feel better about yourself. You begin to learn that not being yourself causes stress and unhappiness. There is nothing more debilitating than not being the kind of person you want to be or leading the kind of life you want to live.

Improving the way you feel about yourself isn't easy. It may be a painful and difficult task, especially if you have experienced deep-seated emotional hurt. But when you have the confidence simply to be yourself, the rewards are immense. All the stress management techniques mentioned in this book are excellent ways to improve self-awareness, especially those that encourage you to relax and take better care of yourself, but improving your communication skills and emotional confidence are of particular importance.

IT'S OKAY TO ASK FOR WHAT YOU WANT

If you can't communicate well this can cause stress. You won't be able to get your point of view across or your needs met. Talking is a natural skill, but effective communication needs to be learned. The following suggestions may help.

- *Listen.* Give others the opportunity to express themselves without constantly giving your opinion. Show others respect, try to understand them and you may find yourself better understood in return.

  When someone talks to you don't think about what you will say in return. Don't advise or criticise. Instead reflect carefully on what they had to say. You might like to restate, reflect back what they said so that they feel you understand.

- *A conversation is a two-way thing.* You also want to be understood. But wait until the person you want to talk to is receptive. If they are not ready to listen they won't hear what you have to say. If they do express a willingness to listen make sure they have really understood what you want to express, so that misunderstandings don't occur.

- *Now and again pause and be silent.* When you are quiet you can reflect. Silence can sometimes be louder than words. It can say 'I'm listening. I'm understanding. I'm there for you.'

- *You need feedback to make communication effective.* Feedback is a good way to avoid misunderstandings. It shows the other person that you have understood. Communication often breaks down when one or both people don't understand each other. You need to make someone aware of the feelings their words or actions have aroused in you without blaming them. For instance, 'When you said that it made me feel angry', instead of 'You are making me angry'.

- *The art of good communication is to understand fully what the other person is trying to express to you.* Use open questions – questions that expect more than a no or yes answer – and avoid questions that are interrogating or threatening. Use questions that facilitate communication, for instance, 'What happened?' or 'How do you feel about that?' and so on.

- *And finally be as honest and direct as possible.* Say what you mean, without causing offence. In other words, be diplomatic. Don't say you don't like the hat someone is wearing, say instead that you think the hat doesn't flatter him or her.

Poor communication skills cause stress because you don't make emotional contact with other people. You go through life feeling misunderstood and alienated. If you find it hard to communicate effectively with others, work on your communication skills. You might also benefit from assertiveness training.

Not being able to communicate effectively puts you at a disadvantage in establishing relationships and causes stress because you don't make emotional contact with other people.

STAND UP FOR YOURSELF

Assertive people relate to others as equals. They know how to communicate effectively without undermining themselves or others. Assertiveness has nothing to do with aggression. Aggressive people stand up for themselves in a way that violates the rights of others and causes conflict. Their manner is intimidating, and they say things such as 'You should, must or ought' or 'It's your fault.'

Being assertive, on the other hand, means you don't exploit anyone. You express your needs and feelings in a straightforward manner. Because you communicate in a straightforward, honest manner, people relate to you as equals and there isn't any misunderstanding. It is easier to be assertive if you are relaxed, calm and well prepared. It helps to be encouraging and as positive as you can when you are trying to get your point across. Use eye contact, smile when appropriate, give and receive praise and behave in a collaborative, not a competitive, way.

You can learn to behave in an assertive way, but it will take practice. Objectivity is important for keeping calm and focused. Keep your request brief and don't get personal. Say how a person's behaviour or actions have affected you, not how that person him or herself has affected you. For example, 'I get upset whenever you do that,' not 'You're upsetting me.' The emphasis now is on what that person did, not who that person is.

Use the broken-record technique – repeating what you want to say without deviating until you are sure that the other person has understood your viewpoint. Try to distinguish between real criticism, which needs your attention, and put-downs, which are irrelevant. If someone is negative about you, ask for constructive feedback.

Your aim is not to win or make someone agree with you, but to find a solution that suits everyone. Such a workable compromise will involve a certain amount of negotiation. Negotiation gets easier if you really listen to and understand what the other party is saying, if you avoid nerves by being prepared, if you keep calm, if you don't criticise the other party, if you keep to the point being discussed and if you are prepared to compromise, take risks, or back down if you have to.

Listen to what others say, try to get your point across clearly, don't get personal and try to work towards a solution that has everybody's best interests at heart.

It sounds hard, but it really isn't. Keep practising and you'll get there. Start with little things, such as making sure the food you order in a restaurant is prepared the way you like it. Don't blame the waiter or throw a tantrum, just calmly say what the problem is and ask for it to be corrected. Throwing in a compliment will make the waiter want to help you. Nine times out of ten you'll get the dish the way you like it. If you don't, take your business elsewhere.

In no time at all you'll be practising your assertiveness skills in more important areas of your life.

DEALING WITH CRITICISM

Criticism can come in many forms, but the intention behind much of it is the same: to undermine you in some way. To deal with this you need to develop skills that help you stand your ground. One of these is not to take no for an answer. Repeat your message, however persistent or manipulative the other person gets, until that person has heard what you say and agreed to negotiate with you.

Another strategy is to acknowledge that there may be an element of truth in the criticism but to follow that up with an assertion of your viewpoint: 'I understand what you are saying but I still feel ...' You may also decide to agree with the criticism, depending on the nature of it, or actively encourage it to find out whether your critic is being truthful or manipulative.

Criticism from others can destroy self-esteem. We all want to be liked and praised and criticism hurts. Much, of course, depends on the spirit in which the criticism was given. If it was intended to help you correct and improve, then see criticism as an opportunity to learn and grow. But if the criticism was unjust, how do you cope?

You may want to bear in mind that unjust or unfair criticism is usually given to make the critic feel important. It often means that you are worthy of attention and the critic feels jealous or threatened. So the next time you are worried by unjust criticism, take it as a compliment.

IT'S OKAY TO SAY 'NO'

You might be able to save yourself a considerable amount of stress if you know how to say no when someone makes unreasonable or inconvenient demands on you. It's likely that you have the best of intentions and are incredibly loving and giving, but if other people are walking all over you, it is time to start practising assertiveness skills. It's time to start learning that there is nothing wrong with saying no.

The only person who has the right to judge your behaviour, thoughts and emotions is you. You have the right to change your mind, say no or 'I don't understand' or 'I don't know' or even 'I don't care.'

If you are helping or being there for others because you really want to, that's fine, but if you are frightened of becoming unpopular or lonely or disappointing others if you stop being everything to everybody, remind yourself that those who really care about you won't put unwelcome demands on you. If you start feeling obligated or guilty in your relationships, then it is time to change the dynamic of those relationships and, if need be, move away from them.

IT'S OKAY TO BE ANGRY

Not acknowledging the way you feel can contribute to stress. Emotional confidence will help you manage stress more effectively. It is the ability to be fully in charge of your feelings and to express the full range of emotions without worrying that you will lose control. Emotional confidence is being aware of your feelings and being able to express them appropriately while responding sensitively to the feelings of others.

Self-esteem plummets if we allow our emotions to 'make' us act in ways that run counter to our values. Self-esteem improves when we are more consistent in the way we react and behave. When you become aware of the influence your feelings have on your reason, you will find it easier to make decisions. You will also have more chances for success and happiness, because you can see the opportunities rather than the problems that come into your life.

Rock-solid emotional confidence is an impossible ideal, but there are things you can do to improve the way you handle your emotions. The first is becoming more aware of your feelings and why you have them.

Many of us find it hard to understand or feel our emotions properly. It is not always easy to trust our emotions. Sometimes they seem so illogical, and we have been conditioned to delay or deny their expression. Yet the very nature of our emotions is to be illogical. Sometimes, for instance, you just need to cry. Stress can be a form of pent-up tension and sadness. Instead of questioning and denying, we should simply allow ourselves to feel what our body and mind want us to feel. Just let worry go in a torrent of tears.

You may find it painful to express your emotions, but feelings, including the so-called negative ones, such as anger, fear or sadness, will lead to improved mental and physical health. This is not to say that we should act on them all the time, but we need to acknowledge that these emotions exist in order to alert us to an area of discomfort in our lives. When emotions are not felt, they cause even greater stress. When they are bottled up, they affect your whole body, especially the immune system, because you are not allowing yourself to feel what is true for you. Emotions are messages that come from your inner wisdom. If they are not worked through, the biochemical effect of suppressing them may cause physical and emotional problems.

Crying and laughing, feeling and expressing emotions, is the only real way we have to acknowledge that our life matters to us. Feeling our emotions shows us how important our life is to us and how important it should be to those around us. Sometimes these emotions will cause pain and distress, but difficult emotions also signal the need for some kind of change in our lives. They require us to act, to change the situation or mind-set that is causing distress, to move on with our lives. Negative emotions, such as anger, are not bad emotions; they are necessary for us to grow, learn and develop.

HAVE FUN

One of the best and most neglected ways to reduce stress is laughter. The positive emotions associated with laughter decrease stress hormones and increase the number of immune cells. Think about all the things you really enjoy doing, and then try to work as many as possible of them into your life every day.

Research is now proving that pleasure does the immune system good. The more fun you have, the more gracefully you will age and the healthier you will feel. When we are happy, positive hormone and enzyme levels are elevated and blood pressure is normal. Even smiling can send impulses along the pleasure pathways to make you feel good. And besides, wrinkles from smiling are far more attractive than harsh frown lines.

Many studies have linked happiness to longevity and demonstrated that there are considerable health benefits in happiness and humour. It is important not only to find pleasure in your daily routine, but also to keep planning pleasurable activities in the future.

This is not to suggest that you treat life as one big joke, but simply that many of us take ourselves far too seriously. Children laugh hundreds of times a day. As we get older we laugh less and less and sometimes not at all. If just the act of smiling can produce demonstratively lower stress levels, think what laughter can do.

Being serious and responsible are not one and the same thing. Laughter and play are cathartic. Find time for them. If you don't have enjoyment, laughter and fun in your life, then are you really living?

In a very short space of time we've covered a lot of ground. You might want to go back and re-read a few chapters. If you want additional information, the Suggested Reading list at the end of the book and the Useful Addresses will help. Stress management isn't complicated. Just take a deep breath, use your common sense, and have fun.

CHAPTER 9

ADDRESSING SPECIFIC STRESSES

In this chapter we'll address stresses related to appearance, money, work, sex, children, religion and relationships. If you feel you are suffering from stress related to a specific area in your life, the following tips might be helpful.

APPEARANCE

Body-image insecurity affects every aspect of our lives and is a major cause of stress, anxiety and depression. The chances are that if you begin taking care of your body with the right diet and regular exercise, you will start to respect and like your body more. But this won't happen overnight. In the meantime you have to stop trying to change your appearance and start trying to change the way you feel about how you look. Have a think about the following:

■ Being thin does not improve your body image. I have spoken to many people who had lost fat or who were at or below their ideal weight who still disliked their bodies.

■ Spend some time really looking at other people your age. Notice how very different their bodies are from one another. Think about people you consider beautiful. Often their features are not perfect.

■ If you think you are overweight, get your body fat tested to see if you fall within the normal range. A reading of twenty-two to twenty-five per cent means you are relatively slender and physically fit. If you are athletic, twenty-eight to thirty per cent is okay.

■ Get to know your body better. Carefully and without giving in to negative thoughts, look at yourself naked in front of a mirror. Counteract criticisms of your body with something positive. Instead of 'I look fat', focus on how beautiful your eyes are, how good your hair looks.

■ Have a good long think about why you want to look different. Why is it so important to you?

■ Listen to your body. Commit to trusting that it knows what it wants. Be honest about what you are eating. Make sensible, healthy food choices. Eat when you are hungry. Stop when you are full. Exercise when you can to help boost body confidence.

■ If how you look is really making you depressed, seek professional help. You need guidance about how to change negative thought patterns and a therapist or GP might help. Call an eating disorder clinic at your hospital and ask for a referral. To keep you on track, you might consider joining a support group that deals with food, weight and depression.

■ Read some books on developing a healthy body image and self-esteem.

■ Try to identify the real triggers for your body hatred. Every time you feel negative about your body think about what is going on at the time. Are you really angry with your partner? Has your boss upset you? Did you feel ignored by the shop assistant?

- Recognise that it is unnatural and unhealthy to look like the models on the catwalk. They are not real people but fantasies created by the media.

- Understand that thinness and youth do not equal attractiveness.

- Separate what you do from how you look.

- Focus on what you are good at. Put your energy into doing things you enjoy.

- A positive body image makes a person attractive regardless of build or weight. Gaining this kind of body confidence starts with treating your body with respect.

- Rethink your definition of attractiveness. Beauty is not about youth and slenderness but about feeling confident about yourself. The sooner you come to this realisation, the happier you will be.

MONEY

There can be nothing more stressful than the knowledge that you are spending more than you earn. Financial problems and debts can make even the most confident among us feel uncertain and nervous. Money can't buy you happiness and self-respect, but financial security can indeed help you feel more confident and secure.

You can, of course, make a deliberate choice not to get stressed about money. This is an effective way to deal with financial concerns as long as you don't lose sight of how much you are earning and how much you are spending. Probably, though, you will find this approach impossible. Your money worries may be minor or major, but the following strategies may help:

- Find out exactly what you spend your money on each week, and decide what isn't necessary.

- Set financial goals for a certain time period.

- Decide what you need to do to achieve those goals – reduce spending, increase income, work more hours and so on.

- Put your plan into action.

- If you can afford it, hire a financial planner to do your worrying for you.

A budget may be all that you need. This means setting up a system for allocating how much money you spend in each expense category based on what you have spent in the past, on your ongoing expenses and on your income. Determine your anticipated income, figure out your expenses categories, e.g. rent, tax, shopping, bills and so on, and determine how much you can spend in each category. Budgeting on a yearly, monthly or weekly basis can keep you informed of your spending habits and relieve a lot of worry.

If you do need to reduce expenses, the process can be amazingly easy. Just review your current expenses. Once you start thinking about your spending habits it becomes easier to change them and to cut out unnecessary expenses. Living more simply and frugally may help you reduce your outgoings.

If you fear becoming destitute, do some research to find out what benefits you would be entitled to. Keep a file of this information for easy access. Think if there is anyone you could ask for support during a difficult time, and maintain strong connections with friends and family.

Setting up a savings plan and putting money aside for emergencies may help ease anxiety about money. Many of us think about saving money but don't get around to it. Yet if you are serious about reducing money worry, putting even a little money aside each week can give you a feeling of security.

WORK

You may be in a job that is stressful, or you may feel that you aren't good enough at your job. You may feel that you will never get another job. A difficult boss or colleagues may be causing you a lot of stress. You may be putting up with a lot for the sake of that essential salary slip.

You can combat work-related stress by really thinking about what you want to do in your career. You might find that further education or study minimises stress and points you in the right direction. If you are tied to a job you don't like because you don't think you are good enough to do anything else, ask yourself one question: How do you know? How accurate is your self-assessment? Self-appraisal is hard to do, but it is important that you do it. List your strengths and weaknesses. You may surprise yourself.

If the problem is dealing with difficult co-workers, don't get sucked into a feuding war. Assertiveness skills will certainly help here and may be all that is required for the other person to back off. If he or she doesn't, speak in confidence to someone in authority about your concerns. If need be, consult a lawyer. Remember too that in some way you might be contributing to the problem. Are you also at times being difficult?

If you aren't content with your job and are suffering from work-related stress, think about what steps you can take to reduce that stress. If you are an employee, here are a few suggestions that may help:

- Talk to your colleagues to find out if there is a problem for them too. Get an idea of stress levels within the company and ways to reduce it.

- Has your company got a stress management policy? Would a stress audit by a professional consultant or in-house specialist be a possibility? If you want to take the matter further, talk to your supervisor, human resources department or trade union representative.

- Delete unwanted e-mails, use the phone instead of calling meetings, arrange video conferencing instead of travel, and during meetings start and finish on time and stick to the agenda set.

- Work on your assertiveness – see Chapter 8 for information on this.

- If you are a manager or employer, before you send your staff to stress management workshops, consider whether or not they are being given unrealistic deadlines and too much work. It's preferable to remove the source of the stress rather than to find ways to deal with it. Remember, a 'de'-stressed workplace has less absenteeism, fewer accidents, better staff relationships and better performance.

One of the most powerful answers to work-related stress may well be increased togetherness and cooperation with others. Talk to the people you work with, involve them and don't get so wrapped up in your own work that you fail to recognise their needs.

And if you don't work, make sure that you love the life choices you have made, that you have friends, interests, hobbies, hopes and dreams. People who love what they are doing have beaten the odds for stress. If you don't really enjoy your life and have at the moment no avenue of escape because of financial or family commitments, for your own sake find an interest that really motivates you. The important thing is to make the most of every day of your life. And if work is a large part of your life you owe it to yourself to ensure that you use every day as an opportunity to learn, to grow, to be challenged and to enjoy.

RELATIONSHIPS

Research has shown that a good social support network is essential to reduce the impact of stress on your life. If your relationships are defined by tension or misunderstanding and you are glad to get away from them, you are stressed out and so are your relationships. In such a case, take things one step at a time. Every effort you make will make a positive difference. Think about all the things that make you feel stressed and take action. For example, if you always argue with your partner or flatmate about who should do the vacuuming draw up a housework schedule.

Ask for help and support

It is not an admission of failure to ask for help. A network of reassuring support from family, friends and colleagues can help minimise the effects of harmful stress. It really is good to talk.

Build positive relationships

Your relationships should not drain you, but make you feel good about yourself. Hopefully, you won't waste time with people who are only interested in themselves or take you for granted. Also, if you believe that friendship is all about your needs being fulfilled, you are not a friend. Friendship is about giving and receiving and is based on the capacity to accept as well as to give love and respect. A healthy relationship with another person adds to your sense of zest and self-worth. If people sap your energy you are mixing with the wrong kind of people.

When you meet someone you feel that you could have a positive connection with, be interested in them, don't criticise but respect their opinions, be there for them and make them feel important. Enjoy their company, but have a clear sense of who you are. Don't let boundaries blur. Don't behave in a way you think you ought to behave. Be yourself. Be a friend, and you will have friends.

If you can learn to accept yourself, you will always be the kind of person people will want to spend time with because you are relaxed, easy to talk to and a pleasure to be with.

Relationships are all about give and take. If a relationship is not making you feel good, and you have tried compromise and communication, consider what changes you should make. We could discuss this at length, but at the end of the day you have a choice: you can avoid the person who makes you feel bad about yourself. Or you can change your attitude towards that person, if you can't avoid them, by reminding yourself that no-one can make you feel inferior without your consent. Other people do not make you feel bad unless you allow them to make you feel bad.

Keeping your intimate relationships intimate

If your relationship is important, you will be willing to put a lot of time and energy into it to keep it strong and healthy. You may want to read books on relationships, attend workshops or counselling. Some of the strategies below might help:

- Engage in regular, open communication.

- Set aside regular time for each other.

- Do something physical together, such as a brisk walk or a football game with the children.

- Be more affectionate. A hug, a pat or kiss can make you feel closer. This may or may not include sex.

- Listen to each other, and don't jump in with your own opinions or try to score points.

- Enjoy silence.

- If you have children, occasionally ask a trusted friend or family member to look after the children so you can spend time together.

- Focus on what you love about each other.

- Give each other plenty of space to be who you are.

- Practise unconditional acceptance and love, but don't ever let someone else try to make you say or do things that you don't feel comfortable with.

- If your life has shrunk to a boring routine of eating, working

other, but that phase didn't last forever. Very few couples who have been together for more than five years still make love every day. The focus is definitely on quality rather than quantity as the years go by.

■ If you aren't that interested in sex and feel that you ought to be, remember that one of the major sources of stress is not being true to who you are. There is nothing wrong with you if sex isn't a priority in your life. Despite what you may have been led to believe, not everyone has or even wants to have regular sex. You are not odd if you prefer going for a jog or having a cup of tea instead. You are simply being honest. And it's the people who can be honest with themselves that tend to suffer least from stress.

CHILDREN

Having children is way up there on the list of life's great stressers. They bring with them great joy, but they also bring great change and that change can involve frustration and resentment. From the moment they are conceived, children have a way of taking over your life. Life isn't about you anymore, it is about us. Here are some tips to help you cope:

■ Stop trying to be the perfect parent. Be yourself.

■ Ask for help if you need it from family and friends.

■ Accept that you will make mistakes and learn from them.

■ The greatest gift you can give your children is your time and your interest.

- Be prepared for your life to change constantly to fit the needs of your child.

If you are a single parent, this brings its own set of concerns, but again there are creative solutions. You can network and gather support from others in similar situations. You can also let go of what others think and focus on doing the best you can to raise the child or children that you love. If you don't know whether you should stay in a relationship for the sake of your children, get involved in counselling and make the happiness and well-being of your children your first priority.

If you decide not to have children, don't know if you want children, or can't have children for some reason, the sense of regret and confusion can be stressful. If this is the case, remind yourself that with every loss there is an opportunity for gain. If you don't have children, you may miss out on the joy and wonder a child can bring into your life. If you have children, you may miss out on freedom, spontaneity and personal space.

LOOK AHEAD

As long as you keep a sense of perspective, it can be helpful to think about ways to protect yourself against the stress of major life changes in the future. Have you thought about how you would cope if you got ill, lost a loved one, lost your job, became a parent, your children left home and so on? By thinking about what you would do in a range of difficult situations, you can ameliorate the effects of stress. Forewarned is forearmed. For example, if your children leave home, instead of focusing on the empty nest you can look for new interests now that you have more time.

BECOME YOUR OWN STRESS EXPERT

You should by now be able to recognise the signs of harmful stress. You may even be able to identify what is causing it and start making positive changes in your life to minimise stress.

And by so doing you are becoming your own stress expert. You become the manager of your life and make changes in your life that can help you respond to stress in a positive way.

You may, however, still lack confidence in your ability to manage stress. You feel that you need some extra help. If that's the case, the next two chapters discuss what kind of help is available. We'll discuss complementary therapies first and then conventional treatment.

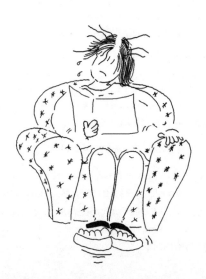

CHAPTER 10

NATURAL THERAPIES

Natural therapies are hugely popular today. Research shows that many of them are highly effective treatments for stress. There are a bewildering number of treatments available and the aim of this chapter is to introduce you to those that are thought to be most effective for stress. Some are simple techniques you can do yourself. Others are more complicated, requiring the guidance of an expert.

In experienced hands, these therapies are safe, but you should always ensure that you find a qualified and experienced practitioner. If you have any health problems or concerns be sure to check with your doctor before starting treatment. Some of the treatments, such as aromatherapy, can make you feel better immediately, but others take time and practice. For best results you should make these practices part of your daily or weekly routine.

The therapies have been grouped into nutritional and herbal therapies first, and then all others.

HERBAL MEDICINE

Medicinal herbalism uses the curative properties of various parts of plants, such as flowers, trees, bark, nuts, seeds and herbs to maintain good health and treat disease. Herbs can be taken in a variety of forms — tinctures, teas, infusions, creams, ointments, or capsules. St John's wort is one such herb.

For centuries people have used herbal remedies to calm nerves and tackle stress. Herbalism is a serious and refined therapy and an herbalist must be thoroughly trained to use herbs which can be potent and at times dangerous. Seek advice from your doctor before you try any herbal prescription, especially if you are pregnant, have high blood pressure or any kind of allergy.

Warning: Many natural remedies, such as herbal preparations, are available at chemists and health stores, but self-medication is not usually advised and you should always consult a qualified practitioner. Make sure also that you check with a doctor that the medications are safe and do not interact with any current medications, especially if you are pregnant or trying to conceive.

Herbal treatments for stress may include:

- Both *Chinese* and *Siberian ginseng* exert beneficial effects on adrenal function and enhance resistance to stress. Research shows that ginseng offers significant benefit to people suffering from anxiety and fatigue. Ginseng, particularly *Panax ginseng*, can restore adrenal functioning for individuals under extreme stress.

  Panax ginseng is generally regarded as more potent than Siberian ginseng. If you have been under chronic stress and constantly feel anxious, Panax ginseng is advisable, but if you have been under mild to moderate stress, Siberian ginseng may be your best choice.

  Many types and grades of ginseng extracts are available, and each individual's tolerance to ginseng is unique. It is advisable to consult a qualified herbalist to get the dose that is right for you. Too much, or the wrong kind, of ginseng can produce unpleasant symptoms and increase anxiety levels.

■ *Chamomile* made as a tea or added to a hot bath can also relieve tension. German (wild) chamomile is the most potent, while Roman chamomile is less bitter.

■ *Kava Kava* is a drink made from kava root and is used in the Islands of the Pacific for its calming effect and its ability to promote sociability. Preparations of kava root are now gaining popularity in Europe and the US for their mildly sedative effect.

Kava drinkers relate a pleasant sense of tranquillity and sociability on consumption and a reduction in anxiety. If you take standardised kava extracts at recommended levels there should be no side-effects. High doses are unnecessary and should not be encouraged. Always follow the therapeutic dosage recommended, which is usually between 135 and 210 mg daily. Avoid if you are pregnant, breastfeeding or on medication.

■ *Catnip* is an effective anti-stress herb that also causes drowsiness.

■ *Passionflower* can calm and relax and is useful in relieving insomnia. It has a mildly sedative effect, like kava and valerian. Make as a tea, or take the tincture (herbal liquid concentrate) or capsules.

■ *Rosemary* is good for stress-induced headaches. It has a mild sedative action and can help with fatigue. Make a tea by steeping fresh rosemary in boiling water for a few minutes, with a saucer over the cup to avoid losing vital oils, or add to your bath. It can also be bought in tincture form.

- *Valerian* keeps the nervous system from being overwhelmed. It also helps to ease stress-related headaches.

- *St John's wort* or *Hypericum perforatum* is a naturally occurring herb that is widely used and prescribed in Europe for depression. It is emerging as one of the most popular, effective and safest antidepressants, perhaps even more popular than conventional antidepressants. For example, in Germany it is the number one antidepressant prescribed by doctors, far outselling Prozac. Every year German doctors write three million prescriptions, as compared with 240,000 for Prozac.

  Research is showing that St John's wort is as effective at relieving depression as an antidepressant and has fewer side-effects. It can also help reduce the symptoms of anxiety and stress. Research on St John's wort is still in its infancy, but recent studies show that it may affect the transmission of the neurotransmitters serotonin, norepinephrine and dopamine, which are thought to create a feeling of well-being.

  The target dose in most antidepressant studies of mild to moderate depression is 900 mg of Hypericum a day, and the Kira TM brand is most often recommended. Side-effects are rare but may include stomach upsets, fatigue and, less commonly, allergic reactions. It can also occasionally interact with other drugs, so you need to ask the pharmacist or your doctor for advice. St John's wort should not be used alongside the contraceptive pill or other medication for depression. It's perhaps best to start with a lower dose and build up, but self-medication is a tricky business. Each person will react differently. St John's wort is being hailed as a wonder drug by some enthusiasts, but it is important not to put all your hopes on one treatment alone and to keep an open mind. Some people don't feel better after taking it.

NUTRITIONAL THERAPY

Nutritional therapy uses general dietary improvement, special diets, nutritional supplements and herbs to cure ill health. Nutritional and herbal support for a person experiencing signs and symptoms of stress largely involve supporting the adrenal glands – two small glands that are located above each kidney. The adrenal glands play a critical role in the body's resistance to stress. If stress is too great, the adrenal glands will become exhausted and not perform well, causing stress, anxiety, fatigue and depression.

Foremost in restoring or maintaining proper adrenal function is ensuring adequate potassium levels in the body – at least 3 to 5 grams a day. This is done by consuming food rich in potassium and low in sodium which should include lots of fruit and vegetables. Foods rich in potassium include bananas, raisins, almonds, dates, carrots, mushrooms, garlic, dried figs and peanuts.

Should I take a supplement?

Medical opinion is divided on the use of vitamin and mineral supplements. Some say that diet alone should provide all the essential nutrition, while others say that it simply isn't possible to get adequate intake through food alone.

Bear in mind that most of us consume a diet that is inadequate in nutritional value. Various studies show that the chances of consuming a diet that meets the recommended daily allowance (RDA) of essential nutrients is unlikely, since most of us are too addicted to junk food. Better eating habits are the ideal, but for the majority nutritional supplementation is advised. This is especially the case if you suffer from stress.

The production of stress hormones tends to take priority over many other functions in the body, which means that deficiency in certain key nutrients, such as vitamin B complex, vitamin C, magnesium and zinc are likely. If you are affected by stress, it is wise to increase your intake of foods rich in these nutrients, but it would also be a good idea to take a good-quality multivitamin and mineral supplement to compensate for any shortfall.

If you do decide to take a vitamin and mineral supplement, make sure it provides the full range of vitamins and minerals. There are thirteen different vitamins and twenty-two different minerals, all important for human function. Make sure that the vitamins and minerals are based on the RDA prepared by the Food and Nutrition Board of the National Research Council. Bear in mind, though, that the RDA are designed to prevent nutritional deficiencies and much is still to be learned regarding optimum intake of nutrients.

Several nutrients are important for reducing stress.

It is well known that during anxiety and stress vitamin C intake needs to be increased. Vitamin C is the ultimate anti-stress nutrient, yet because human beings are one of only seven species unable to make vitamin C, we have to consume it in our diet. When we are deficient in vitamin C our immune system and skin suffer, as vitamin C is necessary to make white blood cells and collagen. Extra vitamin C in the forms of supplements (500 mg a day) along with an increased intake of vitamin C rich food, such as all fruit and vegetables – especially citrus fruits, strawberries, cabbage and broccoli – is recommended.

When people are stressed they often lack energy. The B vitamins are involved in the production of energy. You need to replenish B vitamins daily, and their supply is reduced by refined foods, alcohol, sugar and coffee. You can find B vitamins in wholegrains, green leafy vegetables, liver, dates, figs, legumes, cauliflower, broccoli, salmon, yogurt, tuna and tomatoes. It is best to take B vitamins in their complex form, but vitamin B3, B5 and B6 are very important. Take 50 mg of a multi B complex daily.

Magnesium is instrumental in more than 300 enzyme processes in the human body, including those involved in the stress reaction. Magnesium, along with calcium, is active in nerve impulses and stress-induced muscles twinges and cramps as well as migraines, high blood pressure and depression, which are often related to an imbalance between these two minerals. Food sources include green leafy vegetables, and fresh seeds and nuts. Balancing 250 mg of magnesium with 250 mg of calcium can help to redress insufficient magnesium levels. (Do not take if you are on calcium-blocking medication.)

Zinc is depleted by a stressful lifestyle and many of us are deficient in zinc. Signs of deficiency include white marks on the nails, pale skin, stretch marks, loss of libido, frequent infections and depression. Food sources include seeds, lentils, oysters, wholegrains, seafood, nuts, lean meat and green leafy vegetables. 10-15 mg daily can be a useful boost.

Healing oils

The human body and mind can't function well without essential fatty acids. There is growing evidence that many people, especially women, suffer from a deficiency of omega-3 oils, a type of essential fatty acids. Deficiency in essential fatty acid is linked to dry skin and nerve disorders.

Regular meals of cold-water fish, such as herring and mackerel and seafood, provide enough omega-3, but you may need to take fish oil capsules. Flaxseed oil, a rich source of essential fatty acids, can be found in a health food store. It is best to take the oil in liquid rather than capsule form. Other popular vegetable oils, such as olive, sunflower and corn, contain essential omega-6 oils. Green leafy vegetables are another good source.

TREATING THE MIND–BODY

All the natural therapies listed alphabetically below can be effective treatments for stress.

Acupuncture and acupressure

Acupuncture involves using needles to stimulate points in the body called acupoints. Over thousands of years the Chinese have mapped the network of energy lines that permit the flow of vital energy through the body. In the Chinese system, stress causes or is caused by blockages in these energy lines and acupuncture relieves the blockage by stimulating select points. Those who have experienced acupuncture report feeling calmer and more clear-headed after treatment.

Acupressure is a form of massage built on the philosophy of

acupuncture. In acupressure the acupoints are stimulated to alleviate stress and anxiety. Pressure points associated with anxiety include a point four fingers' width from the inside of the ankle and a point two fingers' width from either side of the spine, just below the shoulder blades.

Alexander technique

This is a system of re-education aimed at helping you regain natural balance, posture and ease of movement and eliminate habits of slouching or slumping. You will be taught new ways of using your body and will learn to think about new ways of keeping your spine free of tension. The Alexander technique can help with stress-related conditions, including fatigue and anxiety.

Aromatherapy

Aromatherapy is the therapeutic use of essential oils that are highly concentrated substances distilled from aromatic herbs, flowers and trees. They are chemically complex and have hormone-like properties; in addition, they contain vitamins, minerals and natural antiseptics.

Essential oils, when breathed in, send a direct message to the brain, where they can affect the hormonal systems, particularly those relevant for stress reduction. The oils can also affect you through your skin if used in massage, a compress or bath. There are over forty oils to choose from; you can either obtain a custom-made blend from a professional aromatherapist or learn about the practice yourself.

Oils can be rubbed into your skin or added to your bath. An aromatherapy massage is a wonderful way to relieve stress. But it is not just the massage that can make you feel more relaxed; many essential oils, such as lavender, evening primrose, frankincense, tea tree, orange blossom, sandalwood, valerain, chamomile and lemon, have stress-relieving properties when massaged gently into the body.

Warning: Ensure that you see a professional aromatherapist if you are pregnant, have high blood pressure or other medical conditions.

Autogenic training (AT)

This system, developed in Canada, combines meditation with positive suggestions to encourage relaxation and creativity. Research has shown that it really can work. The art of AT is learning to focus your attention inwards through a series of mental exercises. These are divided into passive concentration, where you allow your mind to focus on your body; the repetition of certain words or phrases, which induce feelings of warmth and heaviness, such as 'my legs are heavy and warm'; and finally putting your body into certain positions to block out the outside world, such as lying flat on the floor, or relaxing in a chair. The system is effective, but it needs to be taught by a qualified therapist.

Ayurveda

Ayurveda is the name of the Indian science of life. It is a comprehensive health-care system and incorporates detoxification, diet, exercise, breathing meditation, massage and herbs. Stress is believed to be a symptom of energy imbalances, and an important aim of the skilled practitioner is to eliminate them. Yoga can be a significant part of ayurveda.

Chi kung

Chi kung is a form of meditation and martial art. It is a Chinese system that combines breathing with precise movements and concentration with the aim of soothing and rejuvenating the body and mind. Chi kung exercises look simple, but they can be demanding. The beauty of them, however, is that they can be adapted for use by anyone, however fit or flexible. Chi kung is usually taught in small classes and although you will feel immediate results, you need to practise regularly.

The following exercise is said to help you remove stress from your body and feel more energetic. Stand with your feet shoulder width apart and your knees slightly bent. Keep relaxed. Place your hands over your stomach. Take a deep slow breath in through the nose, allowing your abdomen to swell like a balloon. Hold the breath gently for as long as feels comfortable. Exhale, allowing the breath to come out slowly through your mouth as your stomach subsides. Repeat several times, keeping your awareness focused on your breath.

Craniosacral therapy

The skull is made up of plates connected by tiny joints called sutures. The movements of these sutures are minute, but practitioners believe them to be the 'breath of life'. Like any joint, the sutures can become stiff and craniosacral therapists work to relieve such restriction and induce a state of relaxation. This is a subtle, gentle therapy for the whole body.

Unlike cranial osteopathy, from which this therapy originated, craniosacral therapists use other relaxation techniques, such as guided imagery or colour visualisation, to intensify the treatment's stress-busting properties. Mike Boxwell, chair of the Craniosacral Therapy Association in the UK, believes craniosacral therapy to be very effective at relieving stress, putting people back in touch with their own bodies and giving them confidence.

Energy Therapies

Most energy therapies are based on the Asian idea that around and through your body flows an invisible energy that nourishes your body and mind. This energy is thought to be part of the life force, and it is believed to run through everything in the universe. In China this energy or life force is called *qi* (pronounced 'chee') In Japan *ki*, and in India *prana*.

Just like blood circulating, the energy flow can become too weak or too strong or blocked. Practitioners say this affects the corresponding parts of the body and is related to mental and emotional states. Anything can affect the energy flow – the environment, state of mind, diet, exercise, infections, the weather and of course stress. Though we have natural self-balancing mechanisms, sometimes we need extra help. So the aim of the different energy medicines is to restore a balanced flow of energy.

Reiki is one form of energy therapy, where the practitioner places his or her hands gently in specific positions on your body, keeping them in place for several minutes. The effect is of deep relaxation and a renewed sense of trust in life. Other spiritual healers may touch you or simply pass their hands around your body. Spiritual healers believe that healing is being initiated by a higher power, which passes through them to the patient. It is not necessary for you to be a believer yourself, although it helps.

Shen is a powerful but gentle form of energy healing that has had a remarkable level of success with stress-related symptoms. Practitioners believe that all living things have an energy field that flows in certain set patterns. When confronted by stress, whether physical or emotional, the body will go into a kind of spasm, contracting around the pain or emotional hurt. When this happens over a period of time, physical changes occur; the body can't release toxins and becomes tense and stressed. Because the brain is not involved in this process we cannot release the contractions by conscious effort. Only a therapist can release the blockage with a clear flow of energy.

Floatation

Lying in the dark in salted water sounds an odd way to beat stress, but according to some it really can help. The idea is that stress levels plummet when all external stimuli are removed. Floating can promote the relaxation response, since it can be very pleasant simply to lie back with nothing to do but relax.

Flower remedies

Flower remedies are made from the flowers of wild plants, bushes and trees. There is no scientific evidence to prove that these remedies work, but many people swear by their therapeutic effect. There are now more than one hundred flower remedies, but all are based on the principle of treating psychological states. Remedies are taken with water four times a day. The following are some example of remedies:

- *Impatiens* for frustration

- *Gentian* for disappointment

- *Elm* to restore confidence

- *Agrimony* to soothe inner turmoil

- *Olive* for fatigue

■   *Mimulus* for anxiety.

The Bach flower essence called Rescue Remedy is a mixture of five remedies used in emergencies for comfort and calming. It can be drunk in water or rubbed onto the skin.

Homeopathy

Homeopathy is a system of health care founded by a German doctor called Samuel Hahnemann in 1790. He saw in his medical practice that accepted treatments, such as blood letting and the use of strong drugs, weakened the body. Homeopathy operates on the principle of 'like cures like', and accordingly minute doses of substances that cause the symptoms being experienced are administered. A small amount of the substance is placed in the solution. The solution is then diluted and shaken. The more the medicine is diluted, the stronger it is thought to be. The idea is to stimulate the immune system and strengthen the overall resistance to stress.

Finding the precise individual substance required is the art of the homeopath, and the homeopath will also urge you to make lifestyle changes, for example in your diet and exercise.

Although these remedies are available over the counter, you should always consult with a qualified homeopath or with your doctor.

Homeopaths prefer to treat each case individually, but *Natrum mur* is often recommended when a person thinks constantly of past, sad events. *Ignatia*, *Pulsatilla* and *Sulphur* may help lift mood. A special homeopathic combination, *L.72 Anti-Anxiety*, has been shown to be effective in treating anxiety. *Speia* is perfect for hardworking people who do too much, and *Aconite* is good for the highly strung.

Imagery

Faced with stress, many people feel that they can't cope. This naturally makes them feel worse and is likely to become self-fulfilling. 'Coping imagery' and time projection imagery are both effective techniques for dealing with any negative situations you encounter.

Think about what is making you anxious. Then think about the ways you can deal with the situation. Finally, visualise yourself in the situation you fear and gradually picture yourself coping using the strategies you have considered for dealing with the problem. Practise this technique whenever you feel anxious about something.

Or you could think about the cause of your stress and imagine yourself six months later and then a year later. How will you be coping then? Can you see your life moving on? Next visualise yourself in two years time looking back at the situation as it is now. Will it still seem overwhelming? Finally, visualise yourself five years ahead. The problem will probably have faded from your memory. If you find it hard to picture a positive future, imagine yourself with a new friends, a new job or whatever is appropriate to you.

Massage and bodywork

Massage is perhaps the oldest and most influential therapy of touch. It is believed to be very effective in dealing with stress, relaxing the central nervous system, improving the circulation and encouraging the body to get rid of toxins. For instance, a recent study at Toronto Hospital in Canada found that a fifteen-minute massage for nurses significantly reduced tension and improved mood and relaxation.

You can have a whole-body massage, or you can have a massage for areas of the body that suffer most from tension, such as your back and shoulders, or your head. Indian head massage has been used in India as a stress buster for thousands of years. The skull is covered with a thin layer of muscle, which tightens when we are tense. Indian head massage works to relax this muscle, thereby improving blood flow, alleviating anxiety and leading to relaxation in around half an hour.

Meditation

Meditation is a means of controlling the mind so that you find inner calm and can relax; the sort of feeling you get when you are totally absorbed in doing something you enjoy. Unfortunately, it is not easy.

Meditation is a completely different state of mind from that of the normal bustle, and beginners would benefit from a class or a teacher. Don't be put off by the mystic connotations; the technique is straightforward and involves sitting and focusing inwards.

Research has shown that meditation can reduce some of the harmful effects of stress and decrease anxiety and irritability, which are key stress symptoms. People who meditate seem to get ill less and have more stamina and energy.

Most regular meditators aim for twenty minutes once or twice a day. The technique is best taught by a teacher, but you can try it yourself. Sit in a comfortable position with your back straight and your body relaxed. Notice your breathing. Concentrate on the breath as it flows in and out. Feel your stomach rising and falling. Give it your full attention. If your attention starts to wander simply note the fact and gently bring your thoughts back to your breathing. Sit in this way for between five and twenty minutes. Then bring yourself back to normal consciousness, becoming aware of your surroundings. Stretch and slowly get up.

There are various approaches to meditation to choose from. If you learn *Transcendental Meditation*, your teacher will give you a personal mantra or word in Sanskrit, which you use every time you practise the technique and which is chosen according to your needs. A teacher will take you through simple relaxation exercises, after which you sit quietly and repeat the word to yourself. Your first class is generally one-to-one, but after that you will join a group. Sessions last from twenty minutes to one and a half hours.

Mindfulness

Mindfulness is a form of meditation without the esoteric connotations and honed to suit the frenetic Western lifestyle. At its simplest, mindfulness involves stopping every now and then and becoming aware of the moment, focusing on your breathing and gently letting go of stray thoughts and worries. Mindfulness is usually taught in classes, but you can learn the technique yourself. By stopping and becoming mindful several times a day, you will feel calmer and more able to control your stress levels. You can also start your day in a mindful way:

- Wake up a few minutes earlier than usual, and before you move focus on your breathing.

- Become aware of your body in your bed, then straighten it and stretch.

- Think of the day ahead filled with possibilities.

■ Occasionally throughout the day bring your awareness to the moment, becoming aware of how you breathe and getting in touch with yourself.

Naturopathy

Naturopaths are the general doctors of natural medicine. Naturopathy is based on ideas of the nineteenth century European doctors who revived ancient Greek principles of good health based on the importance of clean water and air, good food, exercise and relaxation.

Pure naturopathy or nature cure includes fasting, special cleansing diets and hydrotherapy (treatment with water – for example hot and cold baths, compresses, body wraps and inhalation). But most modern naturopaths use a wide range of therapies such as osteopathy, homeopathy, acupuncture and nutritional therapy. Naturopath is now a term used for a practitioner specialising in medicine in its widest sense, in the same way a family doctor describes a general practitioner of conventional medicine. Naturopaths usually follow a full three- to four-year training along similar lines as conventional doctors.

A naturopath therapist will regard stress as a symptom of an unhealthy lifestyle and will make recommendations, such as taking dietary supplements or herbal remedies, for you to restore your body and mind to good health.

Osteopathy

Osteopathy uses massage and 'manipulation' to correct muscles, ligaments and sinews that have become tense or joints that have moved out of position. This can happen though injury, wear and tear or because of emotional tension. Manipulation means pushing, pulling and twisting different parts of the body. It is gentle and generally painless.

Chiropractors also deal with the muscular-skeletal system, but put more emphasis on the spine. Their manipulation is more forceful and they don't use massage, so may not be so beneficial if you are suffering from stress.

A derivative is *cranial osteopathy*, which is concerned with the bones of the skull (see craniosacral therapy above).

Pilates

Pilates is a form of exercise based on stretching. It is thought to be good for people suffering from stress, as Pilates is based on eight principles: relaxation, concentration, coordination, alignment, breathing, flowing movements, centring and stamina. It is a balanced workout that starts very gently by targeting core postural muscles and results in increased strength and flexibility. It differs from other fitness classes in that the correct posture and alignment of the body is always taken into account.

Reflexology

Reflexology is an ancient therapy that can be helpful for treating stress and stress-related conditions. Medical tests have shown that reflexology can produce a wide range of benefits from improving circulation and digestion to reducing insomnia and stress and regulating hormones. Like acupuncture, it is based on the idea of energy flow. Reflexologists believe that particular points on the feet and hands, and sometimes the ear, are connected by energy channels to different parts of the body. By pressing, massaging and holding the points – usually on the feet – they can release blockages and restore energy flow to the whole body. Whether you believe this or not, there can be nothing more relaxing than a gentle foot rub at the end of a stressful day.

The following can be very helpful for those suffering from stress.

Find the point in the furrow of the top of the foot between the first and second toes where the bones merge. Press gently.

Find the point in the web between your thumb and index finger on the back of the hand, and press gently. Locate the point in the middle of the top of the head between the ears. Press gently.

Tai chi

Tai chi is a gentle art that employs meditation and calm, smooth dance movements to improve the health of mind, body and spirit. Breathing should be coordinated with movement. In order to make a significant difference to health, tai chi needs to be practised regularly.

Yoga and pranayama

Like tai chi, yoga pays attention to breathing and incorporates meditation. Yoga poses keep the joints and muscles flexible, build strength and promote health through nourishing the internal organs with breathing and movement. Salutary effects on the immune system have also been attributed to it.

Yoga is regarded by many as the supreme stress-busting therapy. It is thought to improve a number of stress-related ailments such as tension, backache, fatigue, high blood pressure and heart conditions. This isn't surprising considering that the yoga postures were originally contrived thousands of years ago as aids to meditation. There are many forms of yoga, from the energetic Ashtanga (think Madonna) to Iyengar, with the emphasis on correct form, to the more gentle Sivananda. They all teach pranaymana, breathing techniques that combat stress. For instance, alternating the nostril through which you breathe by gently closing one nostril with one finger is thought to calm the nervous system and bring the two hemispheres of the brain into balance.

If you would like further information on any of these therapies, or others not listed here, contact the Institute for Complementary Medicine (address in Useful Addresses). This is an impartial organisation that acts on behalf of consumers of natural medicine, as well as promoting research into the safety and effectiveness of alternative therapies.

SOME QUICK FIXES FOR STRESS

- Gently massage the point above your nose in the middle of the forehead.

- For stress-induced headaches, press gently with your fingertips the bridge of your nose or under your eyebrows to the count of five, release, slowly press again, release.

- Tense every muscle in your body, starting with your toes, finishing with your shoulders and neck. Inhale deeply, hold for a few counts, then relax totally.

- Kava kava relaxes the mind and body. Avoid if you are pregnant, breastfeeding or on medication.

- *Belladonna* is a homeopathic remedy for restlessness and poor sleep. Try *Bryonia alba* for irritability or *Lilium tigrinum* for moodiness. Available from chemists.

- Set aside a specific time each day to worry, and don't worry at other times.

- Put a few drops of Bach flower Rescue Remedy – a preparation containing various flower essences – into a drink. It's available at any chemist.

- Close your eyes, and imagine you are somewhere beautiful.

- Kneel (sitting on your bottom) with knees together. Let your upper body fall forward so that your face is on the floor with your arms by your side. Relax.

- Drink some kombucha tea, available from health shops.

- Tap the centre of your chest rhythmically using the middle row of the knuckles of one hand. One heavy tap followed by two lighter ones. Do this for a minute.

- With your elbows on the desk, put your face in your hands, cup your palms over your eyes and relax in the dark for a few seconds.

- Shrug your shoulders, tilt your head back and inhale. Exhale and let everything go.

- Put a few drops of orange or lavender oil on a tissue and inhale.

- Roll your head gently from side to side, shrug your shoulders, clasp your hands behind your back and pull the hands away.

- Consciously relax your face. Many of us frown by habit.

- Squeeze a stress ball, available from chemists.

- Bathe yourself in blue light: according to colour therapists this will help lower blood pressure and soothe stress. If you haven't got a blue light, try wearing more blue or visualising blue.

- Pop some bubble wrap. The act of popping bubbles has been scientifically proven to reduce stress.

- Have a mud bath. Mud bath packs are available from health shops.

- Hold one hand with palm up, use the fingers of your other hand to press a point on the little finger side of your arm, an inch (2 cm) below the wrist. Massage in tiny circles for a few minutes.

- Take four drops of Bach Rescue Remedy under the tongue when you feel nervous and stressed.

- Drink a cup of chamomile or lemon balm tea.

- Add three to four drops of geranium, lavender, neroil or Roman chamomile to your bath and relax.

- Take the phone off the hook for twenty minutes, and just listen to your favorite music, have a snooze or read a book. You'll be amazed how peaceful you feel when you give yourself the chance to be alone.

- Have a massage.

- Have your hair cut.

- Get some sunshine.

- Have a good laugh.

- Watch a goldfish swimming in a bowl, or stroke a friendly cat or dog.

- Take a day off.

- Get some perspective. Dr Stephen Palmer of the Centre for

Stress Management in London advises asking yourself what is the worst that will happen if you don't get something done or if the situation continues. Ask yourself how important this really is or if you are making a mountain out of a molehill. Putting things in perspective will reduce tension.

■ If you feel that you are wasting time – in a supermarket, traffic jam or a post office queue – rather than getting tense, use the time to do something else. Gather your thoughts and relax, read a book, phone a friend, daydream and feel refreshed.

■ Daydreaming is what hypnotist Paul McKenna calls a natural stress-busting trick. The next time you feel tense, allow your mind to wander a little and think of all the things that make you happy.

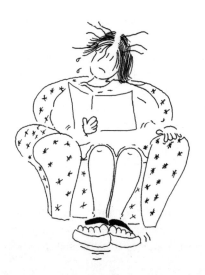

CHAPTER 11

I CAN'T GO ON LIKE THIS

We all sometimes feel that we can't take it anymore. Coping with stress is easier if you have family and friends you feel you can talk to. It is an enormous help if you have someone who will listen sympathetically, offer support and advice if you need it and be there to take your mind off things. Talking to someone can help you see the problem more clearly, get things in proportion and explore all the alternatives.

The very act of reaching out and discussing problems with family and friends can give immediate relief, but what if you don't think you have any close family or good friends to turn to for help?

Loneliness and isolation can be stressful, and fear of rejection may stop you making the effort. As mentioned earlier, it is important that you do make that effort. There are many ways to find new friends through classes, courses, volunteer work, shared interests. It won't be easy at first and you may have to face setbacks, but if you persevere, you will in time be glad you did. Always remember that you are not the only one who feels lonely. There are lots of other people who feel just as isolated and have just as much potential for giving as you do. To find them, you need to come out of your shell.

But if you feel you aren't coping with stress and you really can't talk to family and friends, voluntary organisations, religious groups, your human resources or personnel officer at work, or private or public mental health services may all be places to turn. Details are usually available from your local community health council, citizen's advice bureau, social services department, library or community centre.

YOUR DOCTOR

For most people the first port of call is their doctor. Doctors deal with all aspects of health, but they do vary in their reaction to symptoms of stress. In the UK access to more specialised help can be obtained only through your doctor.

Most doctors prefer to deal with stress by offering advice or counselling. Sometimes just talking to a doctor can offer relief and a sense of perspective to a patient so that adjustments and decisions can be made.

Your doctor may perform a physical examination or arrange for blood tests. Sometimes the signs of stress are so overwhelming that a doctor will need to make sure no serious disease is present and the body is functioning normally even under stress. Whatever the outcome, an appointment with your doctor is a good opportunity to discuss ways to reduce stress as well as where help and further information are available.

Medication can be an effective part of treatment. It can relieve symptoms of stress enough to give you a ray of hope that recovery is possible. There are many safe medications that don't cure the problem but are an effective part of treatment. If antidepressant medication is an option, you will be informed of all the potential risks and benefits by your doctor. Remember that they can only administered by a doctor and a doctor will ensure the correct dosage for you and closely monitor progress on them. You may need to experiment with various drugs to see which one is right for you. The mind is a mysterious thing, and it is impossible to predict with certainty which medication will be most beneficial to you. Don't give up if the first one doesn't work. The next one might. Talk to your doctor.

THERAPY

Psychotherapy involves talking through your problems with a therapist. It is a term used to describe a wide range of therapies and practitioners, and you need to find what suits you. In the hands of a qualified therapist, therapy can be as effective as medication.

Many therapists can help clients suffering from stress, but an unskilled therapist can be dangerous. If you feel you need therapy you are in a vulnerable position, so ideally you should get a referral through your doctor. But if you want to get something organised without first seeing your doctor make sure you know what kinds of therapy are available. Certification and licensing in various forms of therapy varies and it is crucial that you find a therapist with adequate training and experience.

Psychotherapy

Traditional psychotherapy, called psychoanalytic psychotherapy, is the original talking cure. A client sits facing his or her therapist and discusses life problems. Each session takes an hour, and the treatment can last for months or years. It is based on the principles of psychoanalysis, placing importance on a patient's early life experience and exploring their thoughts, feelings, dreams and memories. The psychotherapist's skill is to listen carefully and to suggest new ways of seeing patterns or thought behaviour.

Psychotherapy is suitable for people with stress, depression, anxiety, relationship problems, eating disorders, obsessive behaviour and low self-esteem. The aim of a good psychotherapist is to be a guide and support for you to find your own solution.

Look for accreditation from either the British Confederation of Psychotherapists or the United Kingdom Federation of Psychotherapists. Training takes a minimum of three years. The confederation also publishes two free pamphlets called *Finding a Therapist* and *Psychoanalytic Therapy*. The UK Council of Psychotherapy can inform you about qualified psychotherapists.

In the US there are no rules or restrictions about who can call themselves a psychotherapist. If you are referred to someone who calls himself or herself a psychotherapist, be sure to ask about the person's training to determine if he or she is suitable. In some states social workers are trained in psychotherapy. Check with your state authorities that the social worker is licensed and certified to be a psychotherapist.

One form of therapy often thought to be an effective tool for beating stress is cognitive behaviour therapy developed by a University of Pennsylvania psychiatrist, Aaron T. Beck.

Cognitive behaviour therapy

Cognitive therapy focuses on practical techniques – changing thought processes and behaviour to solve specific problems. It does not try to alter your moods; rather it tries to find ways of altering how you look at things that are causing your moods. For example, you may live in fear of heart trouble and interpret perfectly natural aches and pains as meaning disease. A cognitist, having identified such beliefs, would show you how your thinking is wrong – for example, how your aches and pains can be due to poor posture or muscular strain.

Cognitive behavioural therapists believe that thoughts affect feelings and vice versa. The therapist would use this approach to help you focus on self-defeating automatic thoughts such as 'I'm a failure' and the unconscious belief system behind them. Negative thoughts are analysed as you would analyse the hypothesis of a scientific experiment. They are taken apart and tested bit by bit. Beliefs are explored together, tested and finally changed.

For instance, if you think you are a failure, a therapist may ask, 'Are you a failure in every aspect of your life?' or 'Think of something you succeeded in doing last month.' The therapist helps you recognise for yourself that your thoughts may be illogical, distorted, one-sided and faulty. When you are able to recognise this you can then start challenging negative thinking so that your feelings about yourself improve.

The work you do outside of the therapy session will be as important as the time spent in the session. You'll be given assignments each week. These assignments can consist of listing negative thoughts that occur during the day, reading material about anxiety, reviewing the therapy sessions on tape, writing, role playing and so on.

COUNSELLING

Counsellors often work in clinics or institutional settings along with other mental health professionals. There can be some confusion about the distinction between therapists and counsellors.

Sometimes the difference involves qualification or training, but more often it refers to a different theoretical approach.

As a general rule counselling is shorter term and may be focused on particular issues that have arisen out of the past or present. It can enable a person to find solutions or insights into particular areas of his or her life. Counsellors can be seen as professionals who can help with emotional problems such as low self-esteem, loss, bereavement or addiction. During the course of the sessions a counsellor will help a person look at patterns of behaviour that are stopping him or her getting the most out of life. Sessions are just under an hour long and last for a period of time agreed between the client and counsellor.

In the UK a doctor can give you a direct referral to a counsellor if you need it. There may be one attached to the doctor's practice, or you may be given a list of available counsellors in your area if you decide to refer yourself. Usually counsellors who are attached to doctor's practices will see clients in a room attached to the surgery. You will probably be offered about six sessions. Counsellors who are employed as part of a doctor's or GP practice will have had their qualifications and references checked.

Finding the right counsellor may be a process of trial and error. They follow a range of theoretical backgrounds or 'models'. You may find this confusing at times, but you shouldn't be put off by wondering where they are coming from. At the heart of the counselling process is helping the individual. A counsellor is there to help you look at how problems are presenting themselves and to help you find a way through the difficulties you are facing.

Should you wish to go into longer-term counselling after the first set of sessions, you can ask about continuing, and if you need to look elsewhere the British Association for Counselling has lists of counsellors in local areas. There is also a reference directory on the Internet of qualified and registered practitioners.

Above all, check that the counsellor or therapist you visit is properly trained and qualified. The British Association for Counselling, and also the United Kingdom Council for Psychotherapists, can give further information – see Useful Addresses for contact details.

In the US the term counsellor is used to describe a wide variety of different mental health professionals. Some counsellors hold a C.A.C., which means they are certified to counsel people on alcohol and drugs, but in most states there are no uniform licences or certification required to call oneself a counsellor. Check that the counsellor has experience working with people who are mentally ill and a bachelor's or associate's degree in psychology, counselling or a related field.

TELEPHONE HELPLINES

If you want support instantly, a telephone helpline is a good option. This sort of support is often linked to a particular crisis, illness or issue, and many of the helplines are run by charities or major national organisations.

Not all helplines are satisfactory, so be careful. Make sure they aren't charging for the call and that the calls are confidential. The phone helpers should also be fully trained in offering the correct kind of emotional support and suggesting further treatment. Your local library should have a Telephone Helpers Directory, which lists those with trained and qualified staff in your state or country. In the UK find out if the helpline is a member of the Telephone Helplines Association, an organisation that encourages good practice. You can find the Telephone Helplines Association on the Web – see Useful Addresses for contact details and for a list of more helpline numbers.

One of the most well-known helplines in the UK is the Samaritans. The Samaritans are not just for moments of utter despair: they are also there for anyone who needs to talk about how they are feeling in a safe and confidential manner. In fact, the Samaritans prefer if you contact them before stress threatens to overwhelm you. Nothing is too trivial to the Samaritans. Other crisis lines in your state or county, such as 'Contact' in Dallas, Texas operate along similar guidelines.

If you have never called a helpline, you may wonder what to expect. The answer is that when you call a person will say hello and ask how he or she can help. That person will then listen to what you have to say. They won't judge, criticise, or give advice, and the conversation is in complete confidence. The listener will simply allow you to explore your feelings.

SUPPORT GROUPS

Support groups meet regularly, often locally and often in halls or houses. They are formed around the experience of anxiety or addiction and offer every member of the group a chance to share their experience. Talking to others can be reassuring and comforting. Support is given and support is received, lessening one's sense of isolation.

Lists of support groups can be found at doctor's practices or health centres. Many of the organisations listed in Useful Addresses in this book also run support groups, and you may want to phone them for details. Your library, health centre or hospital may also have a list of self-help support groups in your areas.

SELF-HELP INFORMATION GATHERING

You can gather a lot of information yourself through following some easy leads. Many of the organisations listed in this book offer information or recommend books. Usually they provide this free of charge, although sometimes a SAE and a small fee are required. Your library should have a list of volunteer agencies in your county.

In the US a number of excellent information centres, research institutes and consumer advocacy groups are dedicated to understanding and treating depression. Some, but by no means all, are listed in Useful Addresses.

In the UK the National Association for Mental Health (MIND) offers nationwide support for anyone worried about their own or another's mental health.

Selected books are listed in Suggested Reading, but you can get lots of good information under the medical, health, self-help, psychology and popular psychology sections in your local bookshop or library. You could also try *Books in Print* to track down subjects that interest you.

The Internet is a vast maze of information, some of it incredibly good, some of it downright inaccurate and written by non-experts. Don't rely on it as an accurate source of information at all times.

Useful Addresses lists Internet sites provided by various support organisations that you can trust.

GIVE IT TIME

In this chapter we have considered the worst-case scenario – stress that you can't deal with yourself – but I'd like to conclude this section on an optimistic note: most stress you can do something about.

Time is the most often neglected treatment for stress. Mild stress often gets better in around six to twelve weeks, especially if there is the support of family and friends. Most of the time you won't need to see a doctor or get treatment. In many cases it is only a matter of time before stress management skills yield results. If you can't do anything about your problem, hopefully you can change the way you feel about it and feel less stressed. And even if you think you need to seek professional advice, this doesn't mean stress has won. Doctors, psychologists and counsellors will all be able to help you reduce your levels of stress and anxiety.

It's rare for stress to destroy the quality of your life, but it is common for stress to make your life less enjoyable than it could be. Use the tips and advice mentioned in this book, and you can learn to live with stress successfully rather than letting it overwhelm you.

READING GUIDE AND USEFUL ADDRESSES

SUGGESTED READING

Hopefully this book will be all you need, but if you do want to read further the following will all prove helpful and informative.

Read and learn

Holden, Robert, *Stressbusters*, Thorsons, 1992

Hindle, Tim, *Reducing Stress*, Dorling Kindersley, 1998

Jones, Hilary, *I'm Too Busy to Be Stressed: How to Recognise and Relieve the Symptoms of Stress*, Hodder and Stoughton, 1997

Lewis, David, *One-Minute Stress Management: A Clinically Proven Program for Safeguarding Your Health and Happiness in Sixty Seconds a Day*, Vermilion, 1993

Looker, Terry and Olga Gregson, *Managing Stress*, Hodder and Stoughton, 1997

McMahon, Gladeana, *Coping with Life's Traumas*, Newleaf, 2000

O'Hanlon, Brenda, *Stress: The Commonsense Approach*, Newleaf, 1998

Patel, Chandra, *The Complete Guide to Stress Management*, Vermilion, 1996

Shealy, Norman C., *90 Days to Stress-Free Living: A Day-By-Day Health Plan including Exercises, Diet and Development of Willpower*, Element, 1999

Simmons, Rochelle, *Stress: Your Questions Answered*, Element, 1997

Sutton, Jan, *How to Thrive On Stress*, How To Books, 2000

Tyrer, Peter, *How to Cope with Stress*, Sheldon Press, 1999

Wilkinson, Greg, *Understanding Stress*, British Medical Association, 2000

Wilson, Paul, *The Big Book of Calm: Over 100 Successful Techniques for Relaxing Mind and Body*, Penguin, 1999

Read and laugh

Candappa, Rohan, *The Little Book of Stress: Calm Is for Wimps - Get Real, Get Stressed*, Ebury, 1998

Feeble, Eric, *Stressed Eric's Guide to Stress Management*, BBC Worldwide, 1998

USEFUL ADDRESSES

A lot of information can be gathered from organisations, phone helplines, websites and support groups that aim to educate the public about disorders associated with worry. Here are some of the most well known. Where no phone number is supplied, send a SAE for information.

IRELAND

AA Dublin Service Office
109 South Circular Road
Leonards Corner
Dublin 8
Tel: 01 4538998

Aware – Helping to Defeat
Depression
147 Phibsborough Road
Dublin 7
Tel: 01 8308449

Bereavement Counselling Service
Dublin Street
Baldoyle
Co. Dublin
Tel: 01 8391766

Carers Association
St Mary's Community Centre
Richmond Hill
Dublin 6
Tel: 01 4976108

Irish Association for Counselling
and Therapy
8 Cumberland Street
Dun Laoghaire
Co. Dublin
Tel: 01 2300061

The Mental Health Association of
Ireland
Mensana House
6 Adelaide Street
Dun Laoghaire
Co. Dublin
Tel: 01 2841166

Dublin County Stress Clinic
St John of God Hospital
Stillorgan
Co. Dublin
Tel: 01 2881781

Irish Association of
Psychotherapy
17 Dame Court
Dublin 2
Tel: 01 6794055

Samaritans
112 Marlborough Street
Dublin 1
Tel: 01 8727700

Victim Support
29 Dame Street
Dublin 2
Tel: 01 6798673

Yoga Fellowship of Northern
Ireland
16 Kinghill Road
Rathfriland
Co. Down BT34 5RB
Tel: 018206 31138

Yoga
An Sanctoir
Ballydehob
Co. Cork
Tel: 021 284336

UNITED KINGDOM
Addictions
Alcoholics Anonymous
PO Box 1
Stonebow House
Stonebow
York YO1 2NJ
Tel: 01904 644026 (for local
Helpline numbers)

Al-Anon Family Groups
61 Great Dover Street
London SE1 4YF
Tel: 0207 4030888

Narcotics Anonymous
UK Service Office
PO Box 1980
London N19 3LS
Tel: 0207 7300009

National Drugs Helpline:
0800 776600

ASH (Action on Smoking and
Health)
102-108 Clifton Street
London EC2 4HW
Tel: 0207 7395902
NHS Helpline: 0800 1690169

Carers
Carers Association
Twyman House
16 Bonny Street
London NW1 9PG
Tel: 0845 3007585
Provides support for the elderly
and their carers

Patients Association
Offers details of organisations and
support groups for different
illnesses and disabilities.
Tel: 0208 4238999

Young Minds
102-108 Clerkenwell Road
London EC1M 5SA
Tel: 0345 626376
For parents and carers worried
about a young person's mental
health.

RADAR
Unit 12
City Forumμ
250 City Road
London EC1V 8AF
Tel: 0207 250 3222
For those with a disability and
their carers.

Debt
Citizens Advice Bureau
For local address see your phone
book under C or Yellow Pages
under 'Counselling and Advice'.

National Debtline
Birmingham Settlement
318 Summer Lane
Birmingham B18 3RL
Tel: 0121 3598501

Family Welfare Association
501-505 Kingsland Road
London E8 4AU
Tel: 0207 2546251

Depression and Mental Illness
Depression Alliance
35 Westminster Bridge Road
London SE1 7JB
Tel: 0207 2073293
www.depressionalliance.org

Depressives Anonymous
36 Chestnut Avenue
Beverly
North Humberside HU17 9QU
Tel: 01482 887634

Manic Depressives Fellowship
8-10 High Street
Kingston-upon-Thames
Surrey KT 1 1EY
Tel: 0208 9746550

Postnatal Depression Helpline
Meet-A-Mum
Tel: 0208 7680123

MIND (National Association for
Mental Health)
Granta House
15-19 Broadway
London E15 4BQ
Tel: 0208 5192122

MIND information line: 0345
660163; 08457 660163 outside
greater London; 0208 5221728
London
www.mind.org.uk
Now over fifty years old, MIND is
the leading mental health charity
in the UK. It aims at working
towards a better life for everyone
experiencing mental distress.

Headquarters are London based. See your telephone directory for local associations.

SANE
2nd Floor
199-205 Old Marylebone Road
London NW1 5QP
Tel: 0345 678000
beta.mkn.co.uk/help/extra/charity/sane/index

Eating Disorders Association
First Floor
Wensum House
103 Prince of Wales Road
Norwich
Norfolk NR1 1DW
Tel: 01603 621414

Lesbian and gay issues

London Lesbian and Gay
Switchboard
PO Box 7324
London N1 9QS
Tel: 0207 8377324
www.llgs.org.uk/info.htm

Homelessness

Shelter
Tel: 0207 2530202
London Helpline: 0800 446441

Local Shelter Housing Advice line listed in Yellow Pages under Information Services.

Health

NHS Direct: 0845 46 47
www.nhs.uk
Offers information and advice on whether to call a doctor.

Local Health Information Office
Health Point
Tel: 0800 665544
All health authorities have a health information service obtainable by phoning the number above, which gives information about health problems, services and support groups.

Health Education Authority
Trevelyan House
30 Peter Street
London SW1P 2HW
Tel: 0207 2225300
Provides general advice on healthy living, diet and exercise.

British Heart Foundation
14 Fitzhardinge Street
London W1H 4DH
Tel: 0207 9350185

AIDS Helpline: 0800 56712

Cancer Link: 0800 132905

British Pregnancy Advisory Service
Tel: 01564 793225

Post-Abortion Counselling Service
Tel: 0207 2219631

Stress Management
Local Adult Education Colleges: look
for classes in stress management
and assertiveness training.

International Stress Management
Association UK
Division of Psychology, South
Bank University
103 Borough Road
London SE1 0AA
Tel: 07000 780430
Provides information, advice and
details of stress management
practitioners and trainers.

Traumatic Stress Clinic
73 Charlotte Street
London W1P 1LB
Tel: 0207 4369000
Specialist trauma counselling
services – a national referral
centre for victims of severe stress.

No Panic
93 Brands Farm Way
Randlay
Telford
Tel: 01952 590545

Stress Watch
PO Box 4
London W1A 4AR
Provides workshops and
information.

Telephone Helplines
The Samaritans
General Office
10 The Grove
Slough SL1 1QP
Tel: 01753 532713
24-hour Helpline: 08457 909090
or 0345 909090
The Samaritans is a registered
charity based in the UK and
Republic of Ireland that provides
confidential emotional support to
any person who is suicidal or
despairing. The Samaritans also aim
to increase public awareness of
issues surrounding stress, anxiety
and depression.
If you want to contact the
Samaritans by post or e-mail
write to:

Chris
The Samaritans
PO Box 90 90
Slough SL1 1UU
Textphone number for hard of
hearing: 08457 909192
jo@samaritans.org or Samaritans
Aanon.twwells.com

Careline
Cardinal Heenan Centre
326-8 High Road
Ilford
Essex 1G1 1QP
Tel: 0208 514 5444; 0208 514 1177
Provides counselling on all issues.

Youth Access
1a Taylor's Yard
67 Alderbrook Road
London SW12 8AD
Tel: 0208 7729900
Counselling for young people and
children.

Childline
Free Post 1111
London N1 0BR
Tel: 0800 1111

Rape Crisis Centre
PO Box 69
London WC1X 9NJ
Tel: 0207 8371600

Victim Support
Tel: 0845 303 0900

Telephone Helplines Association
www.helplines.org.uk

Relationship and Family Problems

Divorce, Conciliation and Advisory
Service
38 Ebury Street
London SW1W 0LU
Tel: 0207 7302422

Conciliation Services
Family Mediation Scotland:
Tel: 0131 220 1610
Family Mediation Association:
Tel: 0207 8819400
National Family Mediation:
Tel: 0207 3835993
These provide support for
separating and divorcing couples
so they can sort out arguments
for their children and property.

Age Concern
Astral House
1268 London Road
London SW16 4ER
Tel: 0800 731 4931
www.ace.org.uk

Help the Aged
Tel: 0800 650 650065

Anti-bullying Campaign
185 Tower Bridge Road
London SE1 2UF
Tel: 0207 3781446

CRUSE Bereavement Care
Cruse House
126 Sheen Road
Richmond
Surrey TW9 1UR
Tel: 0208 9404818

Family Crisis Line
c/o Ashwood House
Ashwood Road
Woking
Surrey GU22 7JW
Tel: 01483 722533

Families Need Fathers
134 Curtain Road
London EC2A 3AR
Tel: 0207 6135060
Support for fathers living apart
from their children.

Gingerbread
16 Clerkenwell Close
London EC1
Tel: 0207 3368184
For one-parent families.

Exploring Parenthood
4 Ivory Place
20a Treadgold Street
London W11 4BP
Tel: 0207 2216681

More-to-Life
114 Lichfield Street
Walsall WS1 ISZ
Tel: 070 500 37905
www.moretolife.co.uk
Support group for people without
children.

Parentline
Endway House
The Endway
Hadleigh
Essex SS7 2AN
Tel: 01702 559900

Relate (National Marriage
Guidance Council)
Herbert Gray College
Little Church Street
Rugby
Warwickshire CV21 3AP
Tel: 01788 573241
www.relate.org.uk
Relate has a network of around
130 centres nationwide that
provide couple counselling for
those with problems in

relationships, psychosexual therapy and relationship and family education.

British Association for Sexual and Relationship Therapy
PO Box 13686
London SW20 9ZH

Single Concern Group Support Group
PO Box 4
High Street
Goring-on-Thames
Oxon RG8 9DN
Tel: 01491 873195
For lonely and socially isolated men and women.

Single Again
Freephone: 0800 731 1180

Therapy/Counselling
EAC (European Association of Counselling)
PO Box 82
Rugby
Warwickshire CV 21 2AD
Tel: 01788 546731

The British Psychological Association
St Andrew's House

48 Princess Road East
Leicester LE1 7DR
Tel: 0116 2549568
www.bbps.org.uk

British Association of Behavioural and Cognitive Psychotherapists (BABCP)
PO Box 9
Accrington BB5 2GD

National Council of Psychotherapists
Hazelwood
Broadmead
Sway
Lymington
Hants SO41 6DH
Tel: 01590 683770

The British Association of Psychotherapists
37 Mapesbury Road
London NW2 4HJ
Tel: 0208 8305173
www.bcp.org.uk

Psychotherapy Register
67 Upper Berkeley Street
London W1H 7QX
Tel: 0207 7249083

UK Council for Psychotherapy
Regent's College
Inner Circle
Regent's Park
London NW1 4NS
Tel: 0207 4363002

The British Association for
Counselling
1 Regent's Place
Rugby
Warwickshire CV21 2BJ
Tel: 01788 550899

Alternative Therapies

Institute for Complementary
Medicine
PO Box 194
London SE16 IQZ
Tel: 0207 2375165

Council for Complementary and
Alternative Medicine
179 Gloucester Place
London NW1 6DX
Tel: 0208 7350632

The Aromatherapy Organisations
Council
The Secretary
PO Box 19834
London SE25 6WF
Tel: 0208 251791

British Acupuncture Council
Park House
206-8 Latimer Road
London W10 6RE
Tel: 0208 9640222

Centre for Autogenic Training
15 Fitzroy Square
London W1P 5HQ

The Cranio-Sacral Therapy
Association of the UK
Monomark House
27 Old Gloucester Street
London WC1N 3XX
Tel: 07000 784735

Flotation – The British Tank
Association
PO Box 11024
London SW4 7ZF
Tel: 0207 6274962

National Institute of Consultant
Herbalists
32 King Edwards Road
Swansea SA1 4LL
Tel: 01792 655886

Society of Homeopaths
2 Artisan Road
Northampton NN1 4HU
Tel: 01604 621400

National Council for
Hypnotherapy
Hazelwood
Broadmead
Sway
Lymington
Hants
Tel: 01590 683770

Laughter Therapy
The Happiness Project
Tel: 01865 244414
In the UK, proof of the restorative
powers of a good giggle has helped
persuade the NHS to set up a
laughter clinic run by Robert Holden.

Transcendental Meditation
Freepost
London SW1P 4YY
Tel: 08705 143733

British Federation of Massage
Practitioners
Tel: 01772 881063
For details of a qualified masseuse
or masseur in your area.

Massage Therapy Institute of
Great Britain
Tel: 0208 2081607
Will supply names of practitioners
who trained with the Institute.

The London Centre of Indian
Champisage
136 Holloway Road
London N7 8DD
Tel: 0207 6093590
Offers Indian Head massage.

General Council and Register of
Naturopaths
Goswell House
2 Goswell Road
Somerset BA16 0JG
Tel: 01458 840072

British Association of Nutritional
Therapists
PO Box 17436
London SE13 7WT

Lifeskills
Westleigh
Broomfield
Bridgewater
Somerset TA5 2EH
Tel:0800 980 1774
Source of relaxation tapes.

The London SHEN Centre
PO Box 115
Beckenham
Kent BR3 4ZF
Tel: 0208 6586505

The Shiatsu Society
Eastlands Court
St Peters Road
Rugby
Warwickshire CV21 3QP

British Wheel of Yoga
1 Hamilton Place
Boston Road
Sleaford
Lincs NG34 7ES
Tel: 01529 306851

US

24-hour line: 1 888 8 ANXIETY
1 888 8 269438
Operated by the National Institute
of Mental Health, this line
provides extensive information on
all stress-related disorders as well
as listing resources near where
you live. The service is free.

American Association for
Counseling
5999 Stevenson Avenue
Alexandria
VA 22304
Tel: 703 823 9840

International Association of
Counselors and Therapists
8313 West Hillsborough Avenue

Suite 480
Tampa
Florida 33615
Tel: 813 877 5592

National Anxiety Foundation
3135 Custer Drive
Lexington
KY 40541
Tel: 606 272 7166

Depression Awareness,
Recognition and Treatment (DART)
National Institute of Mental
Health
5600 Fishers Lane
Rockville
MD 20857
Tel: 800 421 4211

National Foundation for
Depressive Illness (NAFDI)
PO Box 2257
New York
NY 10116
Tel: 800 248 4344

National Depressive and Manic
Depressive Association (NDMDA)
730 North Franklin Street
Suite 501
Chicago
IL 60610
Tel: 800 826 3632

National Mental Health
Consumer's Self-help Information
Clearinghouse
211 Chestnut Street
Suite 1000
Philadelphia
PA 19107
Tel: 215 751 1810; 800 553 4539

Depression and Related Affective
Disorders Association (DRADA)
Meyer 3-181
600 North Wolfe Street
Baltimore
MD 21287-7381
Tel: 410 955 4647

American Psychological
Association
750 1st Street NE
Washington
DC 20002
Tel: 202 336 5500

American Psychiatric Association
1400 K Street NW
Washington
DC 20005
Tel: 202 682 6066

American Association of
Naturopathic Physicians
PO Box 20386
Seattle

WA 98102
Tel: 206 323 7610

Association for Advancement of
Behavior Therapy
305 Seventh Avenue
New York
NY 10001
Tel: 212 647 1890

American Anorexia/Bulimia
Association
293 Central Park West
Suite 1R
New York
NY 10024
Tel: 212 501 8351

AIDS Hotline
Tel: 800 342 AIDS

Anxiety Disorders Association of
America
6000 Executive Boulevard, Suite 513
Rockville
MD 20852
Tel: 301 231 9350

National Clearinghouse for
Alcohol and Drug Information
PO Box 2345
Rockville
MD 20847-2345
Tel: 301 468 2600; 800 729 6686

Al-Anon Family Group
Headquarters
Tel: 212 302 7240

Alcoholics Anonymous World
Services
Tel: 212 870 3400

National Association on
Alcoholism and Drug Dependence
12 West 21 Street
New York
NY 10010
Tel: 800 NCA-CALL

American Yoga Association
513 South Orange Avenue
Sarasta
FL 34236
AmYogaAssn@aol.com

THE LAST WORD ...

'Stress is not necessarily bad for you; it is also the spice of life. But of course your system must be prepared for it.'
Hans Selye

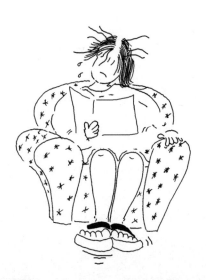